Low Eating GI Made Easy
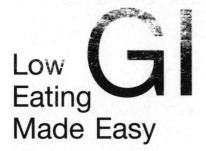

Other books in the Low GI series

The Low GI Diet
The Low GI Diet Cookbook
The Low GI Life Plan
The Low GI Guide to the Metabolic Syndrome and Your Heart
The Low GI Guide to Managing PCOS
The Low GI Shopper's Guide to GI Values
The New Glucose Revolution
The New Glucose Revolution & Children with Type 1 Diabetes
The New Glucose Revolution & Healthy Children
The New Glucose Revolution & Losing Weight
The New Glucose Revolution & Sports Nutrition
The New Glucose Revolution for People with Diabetes

Low GI Eating Made Easy

Dr Jennie Brand-Miller
and Kaye Foster-Powell
with Philippa Sandall

HODDER

MOBIUS

Copyright © 2005 by Prof. Jennie Brand-Miller, Kaye Foster-Powell, Philippa Sandall

Recipe copyright © 2002, 2005 p.155 Johanna Burani, from the book *Good Carbs, Bad Carbs*, appears with permission of the publisher, Marlowe & Company, a division of Avalon Publishing Group

First published in Great Britain in 2005 by Hodder and Stoughton
A division of Hodder Headline

A Mobius Book

2

A CIP catalogue record for this title is available from the British Library

ISBN 0340896000

Typeset in Berkeley Book by Palimpsest Book Production Limited,
Polmont, Stirlingshire

Printed and bound in Great Britain by
Clays Ltd, St Ives plc

papers that are natural, renewable and recyclable products
ood grown in sustainable forests. The logging and manufacturing processes
to conform to the environmental regulations of the country of origin.

Hodder and Stoughton Ltd
A division of Hodder Headline
338 Euston Road
London NW1 3BH

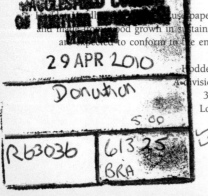

Contents

Part 1

Understanding low GI eating 1

Part 2

Everyday low GI eating – making the switch 33

Part 3

The top 100 low GI food finder   99

Part 4

Low GI eating made easy tables   219

Understanding
low gi eating

Understanding the GI helps you choose both the right amount of carbohydrate and the right type of carbohydrate for your long-term health and wellbeing.

Feed your wellbeing with low GI foods

What we eat has a powerful impact on the way our body functions. It affects everything from our heart and bone health to our skin, hair and even our mood. Low GI foods can:

- improve blood glucose control

- keep you feeling fuller for longer

- help you lose weight

- reduce the risk of developing diabetes, heart disease and certain types of cancer

'JUST TELL ME WHAT TO EAT!'

These days, working out exactly what you should be eating can be confusing. There are so many people and organisations – particularly the media – with an opinion on the best diet, whether it be low carb, low fat, high protein or any number of fad ideas, that wading through it all seems like mission impossible.

Once upon a time it seemed simple – you just cut down on bread and potatoes if you wanted to lose weight. Then they said fat was the problem and you should eat more 'complex' carbs. Now there are the best-sellers telling you to banish carbs altogether – not just refined sugar, but starch too. And we won't even start on grapefruit diets or soup diets . . . So, who is right? What should you eat?

First of all, we human beings are individuals. Being fussy about food doesn't stop with childhood. When it comes to meal times each one of us has likes and dislikes. We are influenced by the traditional foods, recipes and dietary customs of our family background, and, in addition, some of us have special health requirements that govern what we should or shouldn't eat. That's why one diet or set of food rules can't possibly apply to everybody. When you pause to think about it, the one-diet-fits-all notion doesn't make any sense at all.

There are, however, certain important characteristics of the foods we eat that make some better for us than others. The GI, or glycaemic index, is one of those characteristics – one for which we are still learning the relevance to our health. What we do know is that many of the world's traditional staple foods are low GI, which means that they form the basis of a healthy, flexible, diet, whoever you are and wherever you live. A low GI diet is a way of eating long term that suits everybody, every day, every meal.

The fuels we need for good all-round nutrition and wellbeing

You can read this book from beginning to end if you want to, or just flick through and pick up any tips or ideas that take your fancy.

Our bodies run on fuel, just like a car runs on petrol. In fact, our bodies burn a special mix of fuels that come from the protein, fat and carbohydrate in the food we eat for breakfast, lunch and dinner and the snacks we enjoy in between.

Every day (several times a day) we need to top up our 'tank' with the right balance of these fuels.

So, the first step in answering the question 'But what should I eat' is to take a closer look at these fuels – where we find them and what they do.

PROTEIN – KEEP IT LEAN

We need protein to build and maintain our body tissues. Foods rich in protein include:

- lean meat (beef, pork, lamb)
- skinless poultry
- fish and seafood
- eggs
- low fat dairy foods such as cottage cheese, skimmed milk and low fat yoghurt
- pulses including beans, chickpeas and lentils and soya products such as tofu and calcium-enriched soya beverages
- nuts

Protein is also a satiating nutrient. Compared with fat and carbohydrate, eating protein will make you feel more satisfied and keep those hunger pangs at bay between meals.

Meat, fish, seafood and poultry are the richest sources

Protein and GI

With the exception of pulses (beans, peas and lentils), and milk and yoghurt, protein foods such as meat, chicken, fish and eggs don't contain carbohydrate, so they do not have GI values.

of protein. As long as you trim the visible fat and avoid high fat creamy sauces, batter and pastry or crumb coatings you can basically eat lean protein as much as you like – but you will probably find there are natural limits on how much of these foods you wantto eat.

Because your body can't stockpile extra protein from one day to use up the next, you need to eat it every day. By including a protein-rich food with every meal, you can also help satisfy your hunger between meals.

Protein plus micronutrients

Protein foods are excellent sources of micronutrients such as iron, calcium, zinc, vitamin B12 and omega-3 fats.

- Lean red meat is the best source of iron you can get.
- Fish and seafood are important sources of omega-3 fats.
- Dairy foods supply the highest amounts of calcium.
- Eggs are great sources of several essential vitamins and minerals including vitamins A, D and E and B-group vitamins, in addition to iron, phosphorus and zinc.
- Pulses (beans, peas and lentils) are nutritional powerpacks – high in fibre, a valuable source of carbs, B vitamins and minerals and potent phytochemicals.
- Nuts are one of the richest sources of 'good fats' and the anti-oxidants vitamin E and selenium.

 ### Protein: the bottom line

Keep your protein lean and eat according to your appetite.

Watch the fat when cooking. Opt for:

- grilling
- barbecuing
- pan-frying
- stir-frying
- baking or roasting

Be wary of coatings such as breadcrumbs, batter or pastry. You'll end up with something that could have a high GI and is most likely high in fat too.

When choosing from menus, hold back on:

- crumbed schnitzel or rissoles
- crumbed or battered fish and seafood
- meat and chicken pies
- tempura

FOCUS ON THE GOOD FATS

We now know that a low fat diet is not necessarily the only way to eat for weight loss or overall health. Our bodies need a certain amount of good or unsaturated fat (think nuts, seeds, olive oil and avocados) to function properly and thrive. Good fats:

- provide us with essential fatty acids that form our cell membranes
- help us absorb the fat-soluble vitamins A, D, E and K
- form part of our body's hormones
- provide insulation
- help us absorb some anti-oxidants from fruit and vegetables
- help to make food taste better

The problem with fat is the amount we eat, sometimes without realising it. Fat provides lots of calories – more

Essential fatty acids

Your body actually requires some types of fats – called essential fatty acids – which can't be manufactured by your body and must be obtained through your diet. The best sources are:

- seafoods

- polyunsaturated oils

- linseeds

- mustard seed oil

- rapeseed oil

than any other nutrient per gram. This may be great for someone who's starving, but it's a real disadvantage to those of us who already eat too much. The main form in which our bodies store those extra calories is, you guessed it, fat.

The most concentrated sources of fat in our diets are butter, margarines and oils. While it's easy to reduce your fat intake when you can see it, it's difficult with the concealed fats in foods such as cakes, biscuits, crisps and muffins, regular pop corn or a packet of instant noodles. That's why it's important to read the labels on food packaging.

It's not just the quantity of fat in your diet you have to think about – the type of fat can make a big difference to your health and your waistline. Focus on including the good fats in your diet and minimising foods that are high in saturated fat and trans fatty acids.

While a low fat diet is recommended for weight loss, this doesn't mean a no fat diet. Studies show that some fats, particularly those found in fish, nuts and olive oil, are beneficial in reducing abdominal fat when included as part of a weight loss diet.

Health tip:

When shopping, look for products low in saturated fat, rather than just low fat products. The saturated fat content should be *less than 20 per cent of the total fat.*

Choosing the good fats

Emphasise the following mono- and polyunsaturated fats in your diet:

- olive and rapeseed oils
- mustard seed oil

- margarines and spreads made with rapeseed, sunflower or other seed oils
- avocados
- fish, shellfish, prawns, scallops, etc.
- walnuts, almonds, cashews, etc.
- olives
- muesli (not toasted)
- linseeds

Giving bad fats the flick

Minimise saturated fats and oils including:

- fatty meats and meat products – e.g. sausages, salami
- full fat dairy products – milk, cream, cheese, ice-cream, yoghurt
- coconut and palm oils
- crisps, packaged snacks
- cakes, biscuits, slices, pastries, pies, pizza
- deep-fried foods – fried chicken, chips, spring rolls

Fat: the bottom line

Focus on monounsaturated and omega-3 fats for long-term health.

CARBOHYDRATE – IT DOESN'T MAKE SENSE TO LEAVE IT OUT!

Carbohydrate is a vital source of energy found in all plants and foods such as fruit, vegetables, cereals and grains. The simplest form of carbohydrate is glucose, which is:

> **A word of warning**
>
> Some high fat foods – chocolate, nuts, sausages, pizza, crisps and ice-cream – have low GI values. When you are choosing low GI foods, you're after low GI carbs, not high fat foods.

- a universal fuel for our body cells
- the only fuel source for our brain, red blood cells and a growing foetus
- the main source of energy for our muscles during strenuous exercise

So, it *really* doesn't make sense to leave carbs out!

If you were thinking about trying a low carbohydrate diet, here's just some of what you'll be missing out on:

- vitamin E from wholegrain cereals
- vitamin C from fruits and vegetables
- vitamin B6 from bananas and wholegrain cereals
- pantothenic acid, zinc and magnesium from wholegrains and pulses
- anti-oxidants and phytochemicals from all plant foods
- and fibre which comes from all the above, and *doesn't come from any animal food*

 ### Health tip:

Forget about simple and complex carbohydrates. Think in terms of low GI and high GI.

How your body revs on carbs

When you eat foods such as bread, cereals and fruit, your body converts them into a sugar called glucose during digestion. It is this glucose that is absorbed from your intestine and becomes the fuel that circulates in your blood stream. As the level of blood glucose rises after you have eaten a meal, your pancreas gets the message to release a powerful hormone called insulin. Insulin drives glucose out of the blood and into the cells. Once inside, glucose is channelled into various pathways simultan-eously – to be used as an immediate source of energy or converted into glycogen (a storage form of glucose) or fat. Insulin also turns off the use of fat as the cell's energy source. For this reason, lowering insulin levels is one of the secrets to life-long health. However, cutting carbs is not the answer.

What we now know is that not all carbs are created equal. In fact, they can behave quite differently in our bodies. The glycaemic index or GI is how we describe this difference, ranking carbs (sugars and starches) according to their effect on blood glucose levels. After testing hundreds of foods around the world, scientists have found that foods with a low GI will have less of an effect on blood glucose levels than foods with a high GI. High GI foods will tend to cause spikes in your glucose levels whereas low GI foods tend to cause gentle rises.

> ### The 'carb in'/'carb out' balance
>
> The body attempts to maintain a balance between 'carb in' (the carbs you get from food) and 'carb out' (the carbs you burn for energy). If you deliberately avoid eating carbohydrate but maintain your normal activity, you are likely to eat more calories than you need as your body drives you to eat more in search of the 'carb deficit'.

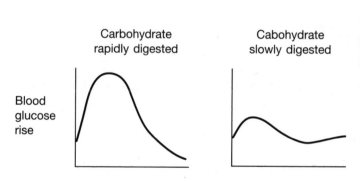

Carbohydrate rapidly digested

Cabohydrate slowly digested

Blood glucose rise

- High GI foods such as white bread, potatoes, jelly beans and cornflakes are converted to glucose quickly.
- Low GI foods such as rolled oats, apples, pasta and yoghurt are converted to glucose slowly.

Our diet these days tends to be dominated by high GI refined and processed carbohydrates – white bread, biscuits, light crispy cereals, crackers, crisps, doughnuts, cakes, and so on. Eating more of these refined carbs means we are eating less traditional starchy foods such as truly wholegrain bread (e.g. pumpernickel), fruit, porridge oats, cracked wheat (bulghur and tabbouleh), barley, dried peas, beans and lentils. These low GI foods are not only digested more slowly, they are also richer in micronutrients than their high GI counterparts.

Carbs: the bottom line

Carbohydrate is the mostly widely consumed substance in the world after water – it's cheap, plentiful, sustainable and the basis for a healthy diet. Choosing delicious, safe and satiating low GI carbs reduces your day-long insulin levels more effectively than any other single dietary change.

Taste test

Try this simple test for yourself. Take a bite of fluffy white bread and keep it in your mouth for two minutes. What's left? Virtually nothing – the enzymes in your mouth have made short work of it. Now take a cooked (al dente) pasta shell (or other shape) and hold it in your mouth. After two minutes, you'll find you still have a clearly defined piece of pasta left. That's because the carbohydrates in the pasta are resistant to enzyme action. So it is with all the starches in low GI foods.

Yesterday, today and tomorrow . . .

About 10 000 years ago, when humans moved from hunting and gathering to farming, our diet was very different from what it is today, and it suited our bodies just fine. We ate a fair bit of meat and seafood, plenty of vegetables and fruits, tree seeds such as nuts and pulses and coarsely ground cereal grains. We may not have had any labour-saving devices, but preparation was pretty uncomplicated – we ground the grains between stones and cooked food over an open fire. This meant we digested and absorbed food slowly and the blood glucose rise after meals was gradual and prolonged.

That all changed with the 19th-century industrial revolution which brought prosperity and radical inventions – and a fundamental shift in our diet. We began to eat much more refined carbs and far fewer beans and pulses. And we tucked into sponge cakes and fluffy white breads all made with the powdery white flour that the high-speed roller mills were able to produce. We now know that this shift has triggered a string of unintended health effects, many of which are beginning to reach epidemic proportions. This new diet meant the blood glucose rise after a meal was higher and more prolonged, making the pancreas produce more insulin.

Traditional diets all around the world contain slowly digested and absorbed carbohydrate – foods we now know have a low GI. Today we eat more carbohydrate in the form of refined sugars, starches and cereal products. These high GI carbs have been shown to spike insulin levels, which can promote hunger and, over the long term, may increase the rates of obesity and other chronic diseases of ageing.

SO WHAT DOES GI HAVE TO DO WITH YOU?

Eating a lot of high GI foods can put pressure on your health because it pushes your body to extremes. This is especially true if you are overweight and sedentary. In the same way that the stormwater pipes of a city are over-loaded after a heavy downpour, your body's glucose response mechanisms are stretched after a load of quickly digested carbs.

Switching to eating mainly low GI carbs that slowly trickle glucose into your blood stream keeps your energy levels perfectly balanced and means you will feel fuller for longer between meals. The whole idea is to replace highly refined carbohydrate such as white bread, sugary treats and crispy, puffed cereals with less processed carbs such as wholegrain bread, pasta, beans, fruit and vegetables.

Only foods containing carbohydrates can have their GI measured. And although the GI applies to the carbo-hydrate, its 'value' – high or low – is influenced by how it is packaged in the food, including the presence of protein, fat and water.

Health tip:

High GI foods eaten with low GI foods score somewhere in between, so there's no need to completely avoid eating high GI foods like baked potatoes. Just include some low GI foods at the same meal. You can live with a low GI diet – it's all about moderation.

GI – whoever thought of that?

It all began with researchers trying to discover the best foods for people with diabetes. The aim was to find out which carbohydrates raised blood glucose the least. Scientists found that when people ate a specified portion of ice-cream it raised their blood glucose just as much as the portion of potato did. Up till then everyone with diabetes was being told to avoid all sweets. Everyone just assumed that 'simple' sugar would raise their blood glucose more than bread and potatoes. These days we know the GI of hundreds of foods from studies all around the world. In Part 3 (page 101), you can check out the top 100 low GI foods.

Not so long ago we believed complex, starchy carbohydrates such as bread and potato were more slowly absorbed than the simple, sugary carbohydrate in cakes, biscuits, jams and honey. In learning about the GI of foods we've realised that this isn't true. Foods such as pasta and grain bread are off limits in many low carb fad diets – but it's precisely these carb foods that fill us up and give us energy. All you have to do is look for the low GI types.

Health tip:

When shopping and planning meals, choose smart carbs, the low GI ones that produce only gentle rises in blood glucose and insulin levels because they are slowly digested. Lowering insulin levels is the secret to long-term health.

Crisps vs chocolate bar

Which is better for your blood glucose? Most people with diabetes would see the chocolate bar as taboo, but by measuring the blood glucose rise after different foods scientists have proved this to be unfounded. Crisps and chocolate have an almost identical effect on blood glucose. *Why?*

The carbohydrate in chocolate is sucrose, which is 50 per cent fructose (which has little effect on blood glucose levels) and 50 per cent glucose (high GI), giving it a medium GI overall. In crisps the carbohydrate is cooked (swollen) starch, which is readily digested to yield 100 per cent glucose molecules. Therefore, fully cooked starch has twice the impact on blood glucose levels as the same quantity of sugar.

WHAT ARE THE BENEFITS OF LOW GI EATING?

Low GI eating has science on its side. It's not a diet. There are no strict rules or regimens to follow. It's essentially about making simple adjustments to your usual eating habits – such as swapping one type of bread or breakfast cereal for another. You'll find that you can live with it for life. Low GI eating:

- reduces your insulin levels
- lowers your cholesterol levels
- helps control your appetite
- halves your risk of heart disease and diabetes
- is suitable for your whole family
- means you are eating foods closer to the way nature intended
- doesn't defy commonsense!

Not only that. You will feel better and have more energy – and you don't have to deprive or discipline yourself. A low GI diet is *easy*.

How do you do it?

Low GI eating fits with the first dietary guideline of countries all around the world: 'Eat a wide variety of foods.' There is a large range of low GI foods from which to choose. In fact, low GI foods can be found in four of the five food groups:

- wholegrains and pasta in the bread and cereal group
- milk and yoghurt among the dairy foods
- pulses (beans, peas and lentils) of all types in the meat and alternatives group
- virtually all fruits and vegetables

This is what makes it so easy to eat the low GI way every meal, every day.

Did you know?

The foods most strongly associated with high GI diets are white bread and refined cereals. High intakes of fruit and vegetables are associated with lower GI diets.

GETTING STARTED ON LOW GI EATING

To get started, you need to:

- *eat* a lot more fruit and vegetables, pulses (beans, peas and lentils) and wholegrain products such as barley and traditional oats
- *pay attention* to breads and breakfast cereals – these foods contribute most to the glycaemic load of a typical British diet
- *minimise* refined flour products and starches such as crumpets, crackers, biscuits, rolls and pastries, irrespective of their fat and sugar content

Did you know?

Processing whole-grains into flour increases the calorie density by more than 10 per cent, reduces the amount of fibre by 80 per cent and reduces the amount of protein by 30 per cent. Refining grains leaves a dietary substance that is nearly pure starchy carbohydrate.

• *avoid* high GI snacks such as pretzels, corn chips, rice cakes and crackers

In Part 2 (page 33) you'll find step-by-step guidelines for making the switch to everyday low GI eating.

Three key habits to ensure a low GI diet

1. If you eat breakfast cereal, check out the GI of your favourite brand – you might get quite a surprise. Most of the popular big-name cereals have high GI values in the 70s and above.
2. Choose low GI bread. Check the tables in this book or look for an accredited low GI symbol on the packaged bread you buy. Ask for a grainy bread whenever buying sandwiches. Steer clear of sweet biscuits, cakes, scones, doughnuts and bread rolls made of refined flour (except sourdough) as much as you can.
3. Eat fruit for at least one of your daily snacks and have a low fat milk drink or low fat yoghurt for another.

Getting familiar with the GI of popular carbs

In the table on pages 17 and 18 you will find some common carbohydrate foods, listed according to their GI value. Take a look to see where your favourite carbs fit on the GI scale.

Where does your favourite food fit on the GI scale?

LOW GI <55	MEDIUM GI 56–69	HIGH GI >70
FRUIT		
apples	canned apricots	watermelon
oranges	cantaloupe	
pears	mango	
peaches		
banana		
For more low GI fruits see pages 107–129		
VEGETABLES		
sweetcorn	new potatoes	chips
sweet potato	beetroot	mashed potato
baked beans		baked potato
BREADS		
wholegrain bread	pitta bread	white bread
fruit bread	croissant	wholemeal bread
		doughnuts
CEREALS/GRAINS		
pasta	couscous	jasmine rice
noodles	basmati rice	cornflakes
porridge		
muesli		
bran cereal		
SUGARS		
pure floral honey	sugar	glucose
maple syrup		maltodextrins
DAIRY FOODS		
ice-cream		
yoghurt		
custard		
SNACKS		
nuts	crisps	
chocolate		

(cont.)

LOW GI <55	MEDIUM GI 56–69	HIGH GI >70
BEVERAGES		
milk	beer	
juice	cordial	
flavoured milk	soft drink	

Note: Some foods such as cheese, eggs, bacon, meat, lettuce, avocado and fish don't appear on this table – because they don't contain any carbs.

GL (GLYCAEMIC LOAD) VS GI

Don't restrict high GI fruit and vegetables, other than potatoes. Because most are not major sources of carbs, their GI is not that important.

Your blood glucose rises and falls when you eat a meal containing carbohydrate. How high it rises and how long it remains high is critically important to your health and depends on the quality of the carbohydrate (its GI value) as well as the quantity of carbohydrate in your meal. Researchers at Harvard University came up with a term that combines these two factors – glycaemic load (GL).

GL = GI/100 x carbs per serving

Some people think that GL should be used instead of GI when comparing foods because it reflects the glycaemic impact of both the quantity and quality of carbohydrate in a food. But more often than not, it's low GI rather than low GL that best predicts good health outcomes.

So what should you use? Our advice is to stick with the GI in all but a few instances. When you choose low GI carbs, your diet is invariably healthy with the appropriate quantity and quality of carbohydrate. Following the alternate low GL path could mean you're eating a decidedly unhealthy diet, low in carbs and full of the wrong sorts of fats and proteins.

You may be wondering what the fuss is all about. Well, some carb-rich foods such as pasta – which have a good fill-up factor – have a low GI but could have a high GL if the serving size is large. Portion size still counts. And while it's true that a handful of high GI foods, such as watermelon, have a low GL, we don't want you to restrict any fruit and vegetable other than potato.

There's no denying that it is easier to overeat certain foods. This is where low GI foods are star performers – the versions with the lowest GI values also have the best fill-up factor. If you listen to your true appetite, you are far less likely to overeat when you are choosing low GI foods.

To give you the easy picture of the glycaemic impact of foods, we have taken both the GI and the GL into account in our tables (see page 219).

> Don't get carried away with GL: it doesn't distinguish between foods that are **low carb or slow carb**.

Avoiding the post-lunch dip

Have you ever experienced what nutritionists describe as the 'post-lunch dip'? It's that sleepy feeling that hits you, typically mid-afternoon. Your high carb lunch and the subsequent surge in insulin levels sends your blood glucose plummeting, driving you out to seek a sweet fix and some caffeine. The trick to preventing this dip is lowering the glycaemic load of your lunch: eat less carbohydrate, choose lower GI carbs and add some protein (such as canned tuna, a couple of eggs, some cottage cheese or lean meat or chicken). And tuck into as many green, red and yellow vegetables as possible.

EAT LOW GI CARBS TO
LOSE WEIGHT

There is no doubt that reducing portion sizes and eating fewer calories will lead to weight loss. Just how you do this is the name of the game. These days, we are eating less fat but getting fatter. Instead of eating fewer calories we are eating more, especially in the form of high GI refined starches and sugars.

Cutting out all carbs is not the answer (remember the carb deficit problem we mentioned on page 9). The real solution to both weight loss and weight maintenance is to be choosy about the type of carbs you eat. Here are some good reasons why.

How do high GI carbs make us fat?

- Eating high GI carbs causes a surge of glucose in the blood.
- Although the body needs glucose, it doesn't want it all in one hit, so it pumps out insulin to drive the glucose out of the blood and into the tissues.
- Insulin switches muscle cells from fat burning to carbohydrate (glucose) burning.
- Insulin also directs excess fuels to storage – glucose to glycogen and fats to fat storage.
- The action of insulin means blood glucose levels begin to decline rapidly.
- The brain detects falling blood glucose and sends out hunger signals.
- Low levels of fuel and high levels of insulin then trigger the release of stress hormones such as adrenalin to scour the body for more glucose. This translates to hunger,

light-headedness and feeling shaky. The only way to relieve the state of hunger is with another snack.

How can low GI carbs help?

If you feel hungry all the time, low GI foods can help you turn off the switch. Here's how and why . . .

- Low GI foods are rich in carbohydrate – an appetite suppressant far superior to fat.
- Many low GI foods are less processed, which means they require more chewing – helping to signal satiety to your brain.
- Low GI foods often come in the company of fibre so they swell and create a greater feeling of fullness in your stomach.
- Low GI foods are more slowly digested, which means they stay in your intestines longer, keeping you feeling satisfied.
- Being slowly digested, low GI foods trickle glucose into your blood stream slowly, helping to ward off hunger.
- Low GI foods help overcome the body's natural tendency to slow down fuel usage (your metabolic rate) while dieting.

The fill-up factor

Can you imagine feeling satisfied after eating just a fraction of your usual calories? Low GI foods help make this possible.

In the early days of GI research at the University of Sydney, we discovered a match between the GI of foods and how satisfying they were to eat. Our readers regularly tell us how easy they find low GI diets because they feel far less hungry. We now know this has a scientific basis – secretion of one of the most powerful satiety hormones (called GLP-1) is higher after consuming the low GI version of your usual bread, breakfast cereal or rice.

Test for yourself and feel the difference

You can experience one benefit of low GI carbs with this simple breakfast challenge. Try out each of the following breakfasts on consecutive mornings, one high GI and one low GI, and feel the difference yourself. By mid-morning you'll be thinking better, feeling better and have more insight into your natural hunger and satiety cues with Breakfast 1.

Breakfast 1 – a low GI option
50 grams (1¾ oz) natural muesli
with 125 ml (4 fl oz) cup low fat milk
and ½ a banana

Breakfast 2 – a high GI option
30 grams (1 oz) cornflakes
with 250 ml (9 fl oz) low fat milk
and a few strawberries

 ## Health tip:

Low GI foods alleviate hunger, making it easier to eat less. Studies show that, on average, kilojoule intake is 20 per cent greater after consumption of high GI meals than after low GI meals.

> ### The weight of the evidence
>
> Studies in adults lasting up to 12 months have consistently shown that people lost more body fat following a diet rich in low GI carbs compared with conventional diets.
>
> In 2004, a study was published in the prestigious medical journal The Lancet confirming that changing only the GI of the carbohydrate in a diet (keeping everything else exactly the same), leads to reduced body fat in animals.

The bottom line: 4 keys to long-term weight loss

1. Choose low GI carbs. Eat regularly and try to include low GI carbs at every meal. This will stave off hunger and strengthen your resolve against temptation.
2. Reduce your fat intake by cutting out the saturated fat in foods such as chocolate, biscuits and crisps.
3. Snack smarter, snack low GI and say 'no thanks' to high GI biscuits, crackers, sweets and soft drinks.
4. Think balance and moderation. Eat a little less. Do a little more.

Health tip:

There's no magic button. It's no secret, either. The evidence from people who have lost weight and maintained it over the long haul is that they:

- Wanted to change their diet to improve their health
- Were willing to lose weight slowly
- Made lasting changes to their diet and activity patterns

LOW GI CARBS CAN REDUCE YOUR RISK OF DIABETES

Did you realise that the higher the GI of your diet, the greater your risk of diabetes? Yes, you read it right. An Australian study of 31,000 people over 10 years found that those who had the highest GI diets were more likely to develop diabetes. In fact they found that eating white bread (not sugar!) was the food most strongly related to the development of diabetes.

Foods with a high GI are digested quickly and cause a rapid rise in blood glucose, and an outpouring of insulin (the hormone that removes glucose from the blood and stores it in cells). If you're eating high GI meals all the time you end up with chronically high insulin levels which could contribute to insulin resistance. This means the cells that normally respond to insulin become insensitive to it, so your body thinks it has to make even more insulin to do the job.

Often, type 2 diabetes is only diagnosed once the pancreas (which produces insulin) is absolutely worn out and cannot maintain sufficient insulin production to normalise blood glucose. Before you get to that point, eating a moderately high carbohydrate, low GI diet can actually improve the function of your pancreas and improved glycaemic control can prevent the onset of type 2 diabetes.

In case you still have your doubts . . .

- In US studies of thousands of people followed up over eight years, researchers found that those who ate a high GI diet were almost twice as likely to develop type 2 diabetes. Interestingly, the effect was most pronounced in those with low levels of physical activity, a known way of overcoming insulin resistance.

- In the US in the past 100 years, the prevalence of obesity and type 2 diabetes has increased directly in proportion to the consumption of refined carbohydrate.

Are you at risk of type 2 diabetes?

About 1.8 million people in Britain are known to have diabetes and another million have diabetes but don't know it, and all are at risk of heart disease and stroke. To find out if you are at risk of type 2 diabetes, answer the following questions.

❑ **1.** Tick the box if you have a family history of any of the following:

- diabetes
- heart disease
- high blood pressure
- polycystic ovarian syndrome

❑ **2.** Tick the box if you are:

- overweight
- over 40 and of European descent; or over 25 and of Indian, Middle Eastern, African or Afro-Caribbean heritage
- a woman who had diabetes in pregnancy
- a woman who has polycystic ovarian syndrome

If you have ticked either or both boxes above you are at risk of developing type 2 diabetes and should discuss screening tests for this condition with your doctor.

What are the key signs and symptoms of diabetes?

- increased thirst
- going to the lavatory all the time – especially at night
- extreme tiredness
- unexplained weight loss
- genital itching or regular episodes of thrush
- poor healing of wounds
- blurred vision

For more information go to **www.diabetes.org.uk**

Did you know?:

Some diet books demonise sugar and advocate strict avoidance, but a modest serving of 2 teaspoons of sugar actually has a GL of only 7.

> A meal with a high GI can result in glucose concentrations twice the level compared with the same amount of food with a low GI.

Low GI carbs – giving people with diabetes a new lease on life

When it comes to diabetes, following a low GI diet can be as effective at lowering your blood glucose as taking diabetes tablets. This is not an exaggeration! A scientific analysis of 14 different studies from around the world of people with diabetes showed that low GI diets improved glycaemic control significantly more than high GI or conventional diets. Improved glycaemic control can prevent the onset and progression of diabetes complications.

On a day-to-day basis, low GI foods can minimise the peaks and troughs in blood glucose that make life so difficult when you have diabetes. Since they are slowly digested and absorbed, low GI foods reduce insulin demand – lessening the strain on the struggling pancreas of a person with type 2 diabetes and potentially lowering insulin requirements for those with type 1 diabetes. Lower insulin levels have the follow-on benefit of reducing the risk of large blood vessel damage, lessening the likelihood of developing heart disease.

The bottom line: the optimum diet for people with diabetes

There isn't any one optimum diet for all people with diabetes. Whether you eat higher fat, low fat, high protein, high carb or whatever, certain characteristics are desirable. They are:

- Eating regular meals and choosing slowly digested carbs with a low GI.
- Including plenty of vegetables and fruits.
- Eating only small amounts of saturated fat.
- Including a moderate amount of sugar and sugary foods.
- Drinking only a moderate quantity of alcohol.
- Including a minimum amount of salt and salty foods.

LOW GI CARBS & A HEALTHY HEART

Eating a high GI diet isn't only related to diabetes. Heart disease is the single biggest killer of Britons and having high glucose levels after meals is a predictor of future heart disease. Sound far fetched? Here's how it happens . . .

A high level of glucose in the blood means:

- excess glucose moves into cells lining the arteries, causing inflammation, thickening and stiffening – the making of 'hardened arteries'
- highly reactive, charged particles called 'free radicals' are formed which destroy the machinery inside the cell, eventually causing the cell death
- glucose adheres to cholesterol in the blood which promotes the formation of fatty plaque and prevents the body from breaking down excess cholesterol
- higher levels of insulin raises blood pressure and blood fats, while suppressing 'good' (HDL) cholesterol levels

How's your shape?

Fat around the middle part of our body (abdominal fat) increases our risk of heart disease, high blood pressure and diabetes. In contrast, fat on the lower part of the body, such as hips and thighs, doesn't carry the same health risk. Your body shape can be described according to your distribution of body fat as either an 'apple' or a 'pear' shape. There are significant health benefits in reducing your waist measurement, particularly if you have an 'apple' shape.

For more information on heart disease go to **www. heartuk.org.uk**

Halve your risk of heart attack with a low GI diet

This might sound like an inflated newspaper headline – it isn't! The results of a Harvard University study of over 100 000 people over 10 years found that those who ate more high GI foods had nearly twice the risk of heart attack compared with those eating low GI diets. This was independent of other risk factors such as age, obesity and smoking, although, surprisingly, in those who were lean, high GI foods did not pose excess risk.

The bottom line: reduce your risk of heart disease

Along with exercise, a diet rich in slowly digested, low GI carbs will reduce your risk of heart disease in several ways. By lowering your blood glucose after meals and reducing high insulin levels, you'll have:

- healthier blood vessels that are more elastic, dilate more easily and aid blood flow

- improved blood flow and less inflammation
- more potential for weight loss and therefore less pressure on the heart
- better blood fats – more of the good cholesterol and less of the bad

LOW GI CARBS AND PCOS

Polycystic ovarian syndrome (PCOS) is thought to affect one in four women in developed countries. Characteristics of the syndrome can include irregular periods, infertility, heavy body hair growth, obstinate body fat, diabetes and cardiovascular disease. In many women it goes undiagnosed because the symptoms may be subtle, such as faint facial hair.

Insulin resistance – where the body resists the normal actions of the hormone insulin – is at the root of PCOS. In an effort to overcome insulin resistance the body secretes more insulin than normal. Among other effects, this leads to growth and multiplication of cells in the ovaries, causing hormonal imbalances.

The problem of insulin resistance

Elevations in blood glucose after eating high GI foods are followed by elevations in insulin. When insulin levels are chronically raised, the cells that usually respond to insulin become resistant to its signals. The body responds by secreting more insulin, a neverending vicious cycle that spells trouble on many fronts.

A low GI diet is invaluable in the management of insulin resistance because it will:

- result in lower blood glucose after meals and thereby
- *reduce the demand for insulin* which can

- help *appetite control* and improve *weight loss*
- normalise fertility hormones

For more nformation on PCOS, go to **www. verity-pcos.org.uk** or **www.diagnose mefirst.com**

Managing the symptoms of PCOS

To manage PCOS symptoms effectively you need to take charge of your health by managing your weight (body fat), making the change to low GI eating and building more activity into your life. The benefits will include:

- improving PCOS symptoms
- achieving and maintaining healthy weight
- controlling blood glucose and insulin levels
- boosting fertility
- gaining control and quality of life

The bottom line: eating well if you have PCOS

If you have PCOS, eating well is not just about managing your weight. It can also improve your overall health and energy levels, and reduce your risk of developing diabetes or heart disease. It's essential to eat in a way that helps to control your insulin levels. This means eating small regular meals and snacks spread throughout the day and choosing low GI carbs. Your healthy eating plan should include:

- fresh vegetables and salads
- fresh fruit
- wholegrain breads and cereals
- low fat dairy foods or non-dairy alternatives such as soya
- fish, lean meat, skinless chicken, eggs, pulses (beans, peas and lentils) and soya products

- small amounts of healthy fats including nuts, seeds, avocados, olives, olive oil, rapeseed oil or peanut oil

LOW GI CARBS & ANTI-AGEING

Scientists are beginning to find connections between high blood glucose levels and diseases such as dementia. As we age, abnormal protein deposits form in parts of the brain and eventually interfere with normal mental functioning. High glucose levels accelerate this process. Indeed, the abnormal proteins are called advanced glycosylated endproducts (AGE for short!).

To get a feel for how this happens, think about the browning reactions that occur naturally during cooking – think of toasting, baking and grilling. When sugar is present, the reactions occur faster, sometimes leading to excess browning, i.e. burning!

The same reactions between sugars and proteins occur very slowly inside the body. Gradually the proteins become burdened by the presence of the freeloading sugar molecules and lose the ability to do their job. When that happens to a long-lived protein like the collagen in skin, the elasticity and natural glow of youthful skin fades. The result: wrinkles. We can't stop it entirely but we can slow it down.

PART 2

Everyday
low gi eating:
Making the switch

Don't diet. Focus on eating well and moving more. Enjoy food and make sure you choose a diet that will give you energy to burn. And remember, we all need to be active. Every day.

The benefits of low GI eating

- You won't go hungry.

- You'll feel better.

- You'll look better.

- You'll have 'energy'.

LOW GI EATING: FOR EVERYBODY, EVERY DAY, EVERY MEAL

We love hearing our readers' stories of how low GI eating has transformed their lives. Success stories like the woman with gestational diabetes who swapped high GI for low GI carbs and found she did not need to take insulin – their stories inspire us all.

These examples and hundreds more have helped us understand what works for people and what doesn't. And that's what this section is about. It covers the sorts of questions our readers and clients actually ask. The answers will show you how easy it is to make simple changes in your food choices that will have a big impact on your overall health – for life.

One of our most frequently received requests is 'just tell me what to eat!'. So, in this section, we focus on food and give you some simple guidelines about making the switch to everyday low GI eating. You'll find out how to:

- put together a balanced low GI meal
- how to eat low GI when socialising with friends and family and eating out
- what to buy and how to stock your larder

Exactly how you incorporate low GI eating into your life is up to you. Some people want to eat low GI foods all the time, others some of the time. That's OK. There's room for both approaches. And in reality that's how we eat, too.

LOW GI EATING – THE BASICS

First let's show you how easy it is to eat the low GI way. There's no specific order in which you have to do things, no strict week-by-week list of diet do's and don'ts, no counting, calculating or measuring. However, there are some basics – daily and weekly eating and activity habits essential to good health. After all, this is not a magic pill. It's an eating plan that will help you nourish your body, feel better and promote optimum health. So, to help you get started, here are the basics.

Every day you need to:

- Eat at least three meals – don't skip meals. Eat snacks too if you are hungry.
- Eat fruit at least twice – fresh, frozen, cooked, dried or juice.
- Eat vegetables at least twice – cooked, raw, salads, soups, juices and snacks.
- Eat a cereal at least once – such as bread, breakfast cereal, pasta, noodles, rice and other grains in a wholegrain or low GI form.
- Accumulate 60 minutes of physical activity (including incidental activity and planned exercise).

Health tip:

Make healthy eating a habit. Here are some tips.
- Make breakfast a priority.
- If it's healthy keep it handy.

- Don't buy food you want to avoid.
- Focus on the positive – think about what to eat, rather than what not to eat.
- Listen to your appetite – eat when you are hungry and stop when you are full (you don't have to leave a clean plate all the time).

Every week you need to:

- Eat beans, peas and/or lentils – at least twice. This includes baked beans, chickpeas, red kidney beans, butter beans, split peas and foods made from them such as hummous and dhal.
- Eat fish and seafood at least once, preferably twice – fresh, smoked, frozen or canned.
- Eat nuts regularly – just a tiny handful.

What to choose?

- ❏ Low GI breads – wholegrain, sourdough and other low GI breads
- ❏ Low GI breakfast cereals – muesli, porridge, rolled oats, etc.
- ❏ Low GI cereals – pasta, noodles, basmati rice, wholegrains etc.
- ❏ Lean meat and skinless chicken
- ❏ Low fat milk, yoghurt, or soya based, calcium-enriched alternatives
- ❏ Omega-3-enriched eggs
- ❏ Olive and rapeseed oils as your main cooking and salad oils

Three tips for making the switch

Here's how you can make it easier to develop and maintain your new low GI eating habits.

Start with something simple

Nothing inspires like success so attack the easiest changes first, such as eating one piece of fruit every day.

Do it gradually

Choose one aspect of your diet that you want to work on, for example, eating more vegetables, and make that your focus for at least six weeks. It can take at least this long for a new behaviour to become habit.

Don't expect 100 per cent success

A lapse in your eating habits is not failure. It's a natural part of developing new habits. Falling over is easy, but getting up and keeping going can take real effort. Believe in yourself. You can do it!

How does your daily diet rate?

Try our quick quiz.

1. I mostly eat reduced fat or semi-skimmed dairy foods. ❏ YES ❏ NO

2. I include at least 250 ml (9 fl oz) milk or 200 grams (7 oz) yoghurt or calcium-enriched soya alternative every day. ❏ YES ❏ NO

3. When I drink alcohol, I would mostly drink no more than two standard drinks per day. (Tick YES if you don't drink alcohol.) ❏ YES ❏ NO

4. I generally don't eat takeaway/fast food more than once a week.   ❏ YES ❏ NO

5. I eat regular meals.   ❏ YES ❏ NO

6. I eat skinless chicken.   ❏ YES ❏ NO

7. I avoid adding salt to my food.   ❏ YES ❏ NO

8. I include fish or some other seafood at least once a week.   ❏ YES ❏ NO

9. I rarely eat packaged snacks such as crisps.   ❏ YES ❏ NO

10. I would usually eat five or more different vegetables in a day.   ❏ YES ❏ NO

11. I use an unsaturated margarine spread rather than butter. (Tick YES if you use neither.)   ❏ YES ❏ NO

12. I use unsaturated oils such as olive, rapeseed, sunflower, sesame, macadamia and mustard seed for cooking and food preparation.   ❏ YES ❏ NO

13. I eat at least one piece of fruit every day.

14. I limit fatty meats such as sausages, luncheon meat, salami, hamburger mince, lamb chops to less than once a week.   ❏ YES ❏ NO

Score 1 point for each YES

What your score means.

12–14   Excellent. It looks like you have the balance right and your basic dietary habits are sound. Read on to make sure what you are eating is low GI.

9–11   It sounds like your dietary habits aren't bad but you have work to do in achieving the right balance and lowering the GI of your diet.

Less than 9   Oops! Room for a lot of improvement here
              – just to boost the basic nutritional quality
              of your diet. So, back to the basics (page
              35) and good luck.

THIS FOR THAT

Simply substituting high GI foods with low GI alternatives
will give your overall diet a lower GI and deliver the benefits
of a low GI diet. Here's how you can put slow carbs to work
in your day by cutting back consumption of high GI foods
and replacing them with alternatives that are just as tasty.

If you are currently eating this (high GI) food	Choose this (low GI) lternative instead
Biscuits	A slice of wholegrain bread or toast with jam, fruit spread or Nutella®
Breads such as soft white or wholemeal; smooth textured breads, rolls, scones	Dense breads with wholegrains, wholegrain and stoneground flour and sourdough; look for low GI labelling
Breakfast cereals – most commercial, processed cereals including cornflakes, rice bubbles, cereal bars	Traditional rolled oats, muesli and commercial low GI brands which have been glycaemic index tested – look for low GI labelling
Cakes and pastries	Raisin toast, fruit loaf and fruit buns are healthier baked options; yoghurts and low fat mousses also make great snacks or desserts

(cont.)

If you are currently eating this (high GI) food	Choose this (low GI) lternative instead
Crisps and other packet snacks such as pretzels, Hula Hoops Crackers	Fresh grapes or strawberries or dried fruit and nuts Crisp vegetable strips such as carrot, pepper or celery
Doughnuts and croissants	Try a skimmed milk cappuccino or smoothie instead
Chips	Leave them out! Have salad or extra vegetables instead. Corn on the cob or coleslaw are better takeaway options
Sweets	Chocolate is lower GI but high in fat. Healthier options are sultanas, dried apricots and other dried fruits
Muesli bars	Try a nut bar or dried fruit and nut mix
Potatoes	Prepare smaller amounts of potato and add some sweet potato or sweetcorn. Canned new potatoes are an easy and lower GI option. You can also try sweet potato, yam or baby new potatoes – or just replace with other low GI or no-GI vegetables
Rice, especially large serves of it in dishes such as risotto, nasi goreng, fried rice	Try basmati rice, Japanese Koshihikari (sushi) rice, pearled barley, cracked wheat (bulghur), quinoa, pasta or noodles
Soft drink and fruit juice drink	Use a diet variety if you drink these often. Fruit juice has a lower GI (but it is not a lower calorie option). Water is best

(cont.)

If you are currently eating this (high GI) food	Choose this (low GI) Iternative instead
Sugar	Moderate the quantity. Consider pure floral honey, apple juice, fruit sugars (fructose) such as Fruisana® or Tate & Lyle Fruit Sugar and grape nectar as alternatives

LOW GI EATING GIVES YOU A HEALTHY BALANCE

Everyday low GI eating is easy. Although the glycaemic index itself has a scientific basis, you don't need to crunch numbers or do any sort of mental arithmetic to make sure you are eating a healthy low GI diet.

By following the low GI eating basics we described earlier (page 35) you'll find you are enjoying foods from all the food groups and reaping the benefits of 40-plus nutrients. You'll also be taking in the protective anti-oxidants and phytochemicals your body needs each day for long-term health and wellbeing.

FAQs about the GI

Are sugary foods all high GI?

No. This is one of the most widely perpetuated myths, even by so-called proponents of the GI – the sweeter it is the more it spikes your blood glucose. Long-held beliefs are hard to shift. In our food finder (page 101) you'll discover many deliciously sweet low GI foods from ice-cream and chocolate milk to floral honey and fresh fruit.

Should I add up the GI each day?

No. In some of our early books we included sample menus and calculated an estimated GI for the day. As our understanding of the GI grew and we talked to our clients and heard from our readers, we realised how unnecessary and misleading this was. The GI value of a food can be altered by the way it is processed or cooked, so we don't believe it is possible to calculate a precise GI value for recipes or to predict the GI of a menu for the whole day. That's why we now prefer simply to categorise foods as low, medium or high GI in most circumstances. We have also found that many people who simply substitute low for high GI foods in their everyday meals and snacks reduce the overall GI of their diet, gain better blood glucose control and lose weight.

Should I avoid all high GI foods?

No. There is no need to eat only low GI foods. While you will benefit from eating low GI carbs at each meal, this doesn't have to be at the exclusion of all others. High GI foods such as potatoes and wholemeal bread make a valuable nutritional contribution to our diet and when eaten with protein foods or low GI carbs, the overall GI value of the meal will be medium.

What's the GI of meat, chicken, fish, eggs and cheese?

There is no point wondering about the GI of meat, eggs, fish and cheese – these foods don't have one. The same goes for most of the vegetable kingdom – foods such as broccoli, tomatoes, pumpkin and parsnips contain so little carbohydrate that their GI is either impossible to measure or irrelevant. But these foods are part of a healthy, balanced diet and we're asked about them all the time, so we have included them in our tables.

Should I be pedantic about GI values?

No. Whether a food's GI is 56 or 64 isn't biologically distinguishable. Normal day-to-day variation in the human body could obscure the difference in these values. Generally a variation of more than 10 could be considered different.

Does a food's GI value make it good or bad for you?

No. When choosing foods the glycaemic index is not intended to be used on its own. A food's GI value doesn't make it good or bad for you. The nutritional benefits of different foods are many and varied. Meat and fish are protein rich, wholegrains are rich in carbs, while fruit and vegetables are rich in vitamins, minerals and anti-oxidants. We suggest you base your food choices on the overall nutritional content, along with the amount of saturated fat, salt, fibre and, of course, the GI value. In the food finder we highlight some of the many important nutritional benefits of the top 100 low GI foods.

Avoid these common mistakes about food and eating

Giving food a low priority

People who give food a low priority often skip meals, grab food on the run, or become overhungry then overindulge to compensate. Usually all three and in this order! Some people take better care of their cars than their bodies. Remember, food is our fuel for a healthy life – we need it to live, breathe and go about our everyday tasks. So schedule choosing, preparing and eating healthy food into your day.

Not eating enough vegetables

Three vegetables on your dinner plate is not enough. You need to eat a variety of vegetables in different forms at different times of the day. When you follow our '1, 2, 3 … putting it on the plate' plan (see page 47), you'll find it easy to enjoy fruit or vegetables at every meal.

Comparing your food intake with others

This is a pointless exercise. First, it's almost impossible to get an accurate picture of what other people really eat (they lie). Secondly, food requirements vary so much between people. Gender, size, activity and age all come into play along with a range of individual factors. Some lucky people just need to eat more than others.

Going on a restrictive diet

If you want to lose body fat and keep it off, restrictive dieting isn't the answer. This kind of dieting that has you obsessively counting calories and cutting out whole food groups is almost impossible to stick to in the long term and can set you on the dreaded 'yo yo' dieting cycle. Instead of trying to control every urge to sneak a morsel of chocolate or feeling guilty when you fall off the dieting wagon, give yourself a treat and enjoy a regular splurge. It's a more sensible approach to eating – and living.

The only way to lose weight and body fat permanently is to change your eating habits and include regular physical activity in your day. We know this can mean changing the habits of a lifetime. We know this is hard. That's why we suggest you make gradual changes, one step at a time, that fit in with your way of living and that you can maintain for life.

Filling the shopping trolley with 'fat-free' foods

Low fat or no fat is a recent trend in food manufacturing. But '99% fat free' doesn't mean calorie free; all too often much of it is high GI and will still cause weight gain if eaten to excess. Here's an example. Take a regular 100 ml/50 gram (3½ fl oz/1¾ oz) scoop of vanilla ice-cream:

- regular ice-cream (10% fat) = 375 kJ/90 Kcal (average)
- reduced fat ice-cream (6.5% fat) = 355 kJ/85 Kcal (average)
- low fat ice-cream (less than 4% fat) = 295 kJ/70 Kcal (average)

So, enjoy a scoop of low fat ice-cream, but say 'no thanks' to seconds.

Health tip:

Commit time to being more active. This is just as important as committing to three meals a day, or substituting low GI for high. In our modern lifestyle, exercise seldom just happens. Like anything else that we want to do, we have to plan it and allocate time for it. It's not 'optional'.

Food minus exercise = fat

SIMPLE STEPS TO DEVELOPING GOOD EATING HABITS

Listen to your appetite

Eat when you are hungry and put your knife and fork down when you are full (not stuffed). If you have a tendency to overeat, serve food in the kitchen and bring it to the table to remove the temptation of helping yourself to seconds and thirds at the table. Also, be aware that we all have 'hungry days', so it's quite normal to eat more on some days and less on others.

Watch for signs of non-hungry eating

It's also normal to reach for food when you are tired, bored or stressed. We call this 'non-hungry eating'. It isn't wrong, but it tends to contribute to overeating. If you are aware of it, you can do something about it – such as drink a glass of water or make yourself busy.

Think about what to eat, rather than what not to eat

Be positive. Make planning and preparing meals fun. Our food finder on page 101 is packed with hundreds of delicious foods, meal ideas and recipes you can enjoy every day.

Eat regularly

Remember the basics: three meals a day is a must. It's probably easier to stick to regular meal and snack times to start with, too. So make meals a time to relax and enjoy food whether you are on your own or with family or friends – you are more likely to feel satisfied if you do.

If it's healthy, keep it handy

Stock your cupboards and fridge with healthy low GI foods and snacks. Increase your chances of eating them by keeping them handy!

Keep occasional foods out of sight

Make overeating as hard as possible by putting occasional and treat foods well out of sight, preferably out of easy reach.

Health tip:

Low GI foods can form the basis of a healthy and flexible diet whoever you are and wherever you live.

1, 2, 3 . . . PUTTING IT ON THE PLATE

Main meals for most Britons consist of some sort of meat (or chicken or fish) with vegetables and potato (or rice or pasta). This is a good start and a little fine-tuning will ensure a healthy, balanced meal. All you need to do is adjust your proportions to match our 'plate'. Here are the three simple steps to put together a balanced low GI meal.

1 is for carb

It's an essential, although sometimes forgotten part of a balanced meal. What do you feel like? A grain like rice, barley or cracked wheat? Pasta, noodles or bean vermicelli? Or perhaps a high carb vegetable like sweetcorn, sweet potato or pulses such as beans, peas and lentils? Include at least one low GI carb per meal.

2 is for protein

Include some protein at each meal. It lowers the glycaemic load by replacing some of the carbohydrate – not all! It also helps satisfy the appetite.

3 is for fruit and vegetables

This is the part we often go without. If anything it should have the highest priority in a meal, but a meal based solely on fruit and low carb vegetables won't be sustaining for long. A plain salad sandwich is a recipe for hunger.

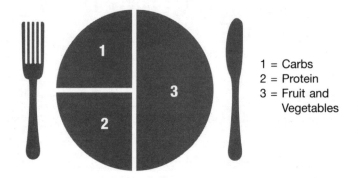

1 = Carbs
2 = Protein
3 = Fruit and
     Vegetables

The plate model is adaptable to any serving sizes.

- As long as you keep food to the proportions shown here, the meal will be balanced.
- As long as the types of food you choose fit within the guidelines for healthy eating, then you should have a healthy diet overall.

Health tip:

Choose healthy foods that you like eating – put them together to make balanced, low GI meals.

BREAKFASTS THAT SUSTAIN YOU THROUGH THE MORNING

No doubt you know it's a good idea to eat breakfast if you want to keep healthy, but did you realise that your food choices may also be a critical factor? Firing up your engine with high GI crispy flakes or soft, light toast provides a short-lived fuel supply that will send you in search of a top-up within a few hours. If you want something to nourish your body and sustain you right through the morning, follow our breakfast basics.

Breakfast basics

Choose foods from each group – carbohydrate, protein and fruit and vegetables.

1. **Carbohydrate** – breakfast cereal, bread, baked beans
3. **Protein** – low fat milk, calcium-enriched soya milk, low fat yoghurt, eggs, tofu, lean ham or bacon, sardines or a little cheese
3. **Fruit and vegetables** – the choice is yours, fresh, frozen or canned fruit and vegetables, dried fruit, fruit or vegetable juice

Eating breakfast can improve:

- speed in short-term memory tests
- alertness, which may help with memory and learning
- mood, calmness and reduce feeling of stress

Breakfast also helps schoolchildren do better in creativity tests.

Health tip:

A healthy breakfast including wholegrains and fruit is a great start in meeting your daily fibre intake.

Seven everyday low GI breakfasts

Kaye's Favourite Breakfast

1. **Carbohydrate**: natural muesli
2. **Protein**: skimmed milk, low fat natural yoghurt
3 **Fruit**: strawberries

Add a little skimmed milk to a big bowl of natural muesli to moisten, plus a generous dollop of low fat natural yoghurt. Top with a handful of chopped strawberries (or any other fruit).

Creamy Porridge

1. **Carbohydrate**: rolled oats
2. **Protein**: skimmed milk
3. **Fruit**: raisins, honey

Cook traditional rolled oats according to the packet instructions in skimmed milk to make a creamier porridge. Serve topped with a scattering of raisins and a drizzle of honey.

Fruit Toast with Ricotta and Pear

1. **Carbohydrate**: dense fruit and nut bread
2. **Protein**: reduced fat ricotta cheese
3. **Fruit**: pear

Spread thick slices of a dense fruit and nut bread with reduced fat ricotta cheese and top with sliced fresh pear (peeled if you prefer). Sprinkle with cinnamon sugar to serve.

Eggs with Mushrooms and Parsley

1. **Carbohydrate**: soya and linseed bread
2　**Protein**: eggs
3　**Vegetables**: mushrooms, parsley

Slice a generous handful of button mushrooms and cook in a little olive oil. When softened, add some fresh chopped parsley and season with salt and pepper if desired. Serve on toasted soya and linseed bread with poached or scrambled eggs. A grilled tomato alongside makes this breakfast extra tasty.

Oats with Apple, Raisins and Almonds

1. **Carbohydrate**: rolled oats
2. **Protein**: skimmed milk
3. **Fruit and nuts**: apple, raisins, almonds

Soak traditional rolled oats in skimmed milk in the refrigerator overnight. Next morning add 1 grated Granny Smith apple, a small handful of raisins and a sprinkle of slivered almonds, stir and serve.

Smoothie 'On the Go'

1. **Carbohydrate**: processed bran cereal
2　**Protein**: semi-skimmed milk, low fat yoghurt
3. **Fruit**: banana, honey

Combine 1 banana, 1 tablespoon of bran cereal, 250 ml (9 fl oz) of low fat milk, 2 teaspoons of honey and 100 grams (31/2 oz) of low fat yoghurt in a blender. Blend until smooth and thick.

> **Did you know?**
>
> Highly processed breakfast cereals are some of the highest GI foods and cost a lot more than traditional cereal grains such as porridge.

Lazy Weekend French Toast

1. Carbohydrate: sourdough bread
2. Protein: eggs, skimmed milk
3 Fruit: pear or apple

Beat together 2 eggs, 60 ml (2 fl oz) of skimmed milk and 1 teaspoon of pure vanilla extract. Dip 4 thick slices of sourdough bread in the egg mixture, then cook over medium heat in a lightly greased non-stick frypan for 2–3 minutes on each side until golden. Serve topped with pan-fried pear or apple slices and a sprinkling of cinnamon.

LIGHT & LOW, THE SMART CARB LUNCH

It is important to take a break and refuel properly at lunchtime. A healthy low GI lunch will help maintain energy levels and concentration throughout the after-noon and reduce the temptation to snack on something indulgent later in the day. It does not need to be a big meal. In fact, if you find yourself feeling sleepy in the afternoon, cut back on the carbs and boost the protein and light vegetables at lunchtime. (Of course a cup of coffee may help too!). Try these light meal suggestions for lunch – or for dinner if you prefer to eat your main meal at lunchtime.

Lunch and light meal basics

Choose a food or foods from each group – carbs, protein and fruit and vegetables.

1. Start with a low GI carb such as wholegrain or sourdough bread, pasta, noodles, sweetcorn or canned mixed beans.
2. Add some protein such as fresh or canned salmon or tuna, lean meat, sliced chicken, reduced fat cheese or egg.
3. Plus vegetables or salad to help fill you up. A large salad made with a variety of vegetables would be ideal. Round off the meal with fruit.

Seven everyday low GI lunches and light meals

Minestrone and Toast

1. Carbohydrate: beans, pasta, sweet potato, barley, rice, low GI bread
2. Protein: Parmesan, beans
3. Vegetables: tomato, carrots, onion, celery and other soup vegetables

When making minestrone yourself or buying it ready-made, choose a filling combination that includes pulses (beans, peas and lentils) and plenty of chopped vegetables. Serve topped with some freshly shaved Parmesan and enjoy with low GI toast or a crusty grainy roll.

Health tip:

Of all foods eaten by populations around the world, pulses (beans, peas and lentils) are associated with the longest lifespan. Aim to include them at least twice a week.

Tasty soups for light meals and lunches

- lentil and spinach soup
- split pea and ham soup
- chicken and sweetcorn soup
- long or short soup with noodles and tofu
- bean soup
- tom yum soup
- pumpkin soup
- mushroom soup

> ## Pulses
>
> Versatile, filling, nutritious beans, peas and lentils are low in calories and provide a valuable source of protein and carbs, which is why we include them as both a carb and protein food in our ingredient listing.

Snack Bar Sandwich

1. **Carbohydrate**: mixed grain, soya and linseed or seeded bread
2. **Protein**: canned salmon, tuna or hardboiled egg
3. **Vegetables**: tomato, sprouts, grated carrot, finely sliced onion rings, mixed salad greens

Try a smear of mayonnaise on the bread instead of margarine.

Lebanese Roll-ups

1. **Carbohydrate**: wholemeal flatbread, hummous
2. **Protein**: reduced fat cheese, hummous
3. **Vegetables**: tabbouleh, shredded lettuce

Spread flatbread with hummous, roll up around a filling of tabbouleh and shredded lettuce sprinkled with grated cheese and warm through in a sandwich press.

Mexican Bean Tortilla

1. **Carbohydrate**: Mexican beans (red kidney beans in a tomato and mild chilli sauce), corn tortilla
2. **Protein**: reduced fat cheese, red kidney beans
3 **Vegetables**: avocado, shredded lettuce, sliced tomato

Warm about 75 grams (2½ oz) of beans and serve in a corn tortilla with 2–3 avocado slices, lots of shredded lettuce, tomato slices and grated reduced fat cheese.

Simple Long Soup

1. Carbohydrate: vermicelli noodles, creamed sweetcorn
2. Protein: chicken stock, chicken, egg
3. Vegetables: carrot, shallots

Bring 500 ml (17 fl oz) of chicken stock to the boil, add a handful of dry vermicelli noodles and 1 finely diced carrot. Cook the noodles and carrot for 3–4 minutes then stir in 125 grams (4½ oz) of creamed sweetcorn, strips of cooked chicken (a great way to use leftovers) and chopped shallots. Heat through. Beat 1 egg and slowly pour it into the boiling soup in a thin stream, stirring quickly.

Frittata

1. Carbohydrate: sweet potato, sweetcorn kernels
2. Protein: egg, skimmed milk, lean ham, reduced fat cheese
3. Vegetables: courgette, red and green peppers, tomato, onion, mushroom, shallots and parsley

Stir-fry about 200 grams (7 oz) of chopped vegetables with 2 slices of chopped ham in a little oil until soft. Beat 2 eggs with 125 ml (4 fl oz) of skimmed milk and season with freshly ground black pepper and 1 tablespoon of chopped parsley. Pour the egg mixture over the vegetables and cook over a low heat (preferably covered) until set. Sprinkle a little grated cheese over the top and brown under a hot grill.

Salmon Salad with Chilli Dressing

1. Carbohydrate: sourdough or wholegrain bread
2. Protein: red salmon
3. Vegetables: cherry tomatoes, red onion, red and yellow peppers, mixed salad and baby spinach leaves

Combine 1 small can of red salmon (drained and flaked) with ½ punnet of cherry tomatoes, slices of red onion, red and yellow pepper strips and mixed salad and baby spinach leaves. Toss in a chilli dressing made from olive oil, lemon juice and minced chilli and serve with bread or a crusty roll.

TAKE TIME OVER ONE MAIN MEAL EVERY DAY

What to make for dinner is the perennial question. Most people know that eating well is important, but it can be hard to get motivated to cook at the end of a long day. You don't have to spend hours preparing. If your cupboards and refrigerator are stocked with the right foods, you should be able to put a meal together in under 30 minutes.

Involve everybody at mealtimes

When you can, involve everybody in the household in choosing and preparing meals. Even if you love cooking, it's fun having an offsider – someone to spin the lettuce, turn the meat, set the table, or simply chat to while you chop or stir, etc. It's also a great opportunity to find out about what's happening in other family members' lives! Lots of our readers say they hate cooking, but preparing and cooking meals is an integral part of healthy eating. Easy meals for family and friends can revolve around platters of foods on the table from which everyone can serve themselves. This avoids any complaints about being served foods they don't like.

If you live alone . . .

If you live alone, why not prepare food for two and put a meal away for another night? To avoid overeating on the night you cook, divide up all the food before you sit down to eat. Make use of partially prepared convenience foods such as chopped salads, filled pastas and frozen mixed vegetables to make meal preparation a little easier.

If you like using frozen meals, choose a low fat type and add your own cooked vegetables to bulk it out. Make a point of taking time over your meal and enjoy what you're eating. Don't gulp it down without thinking in front of the television – you can end up eating more than you should. The experts have even given this habit a name: 'mindless eating'.

Eating together as a family not only improves relation-ships but eating habits, too. In a recent study, researchers found that children who regularly ate dinner at home had:

- higher intakes of fruit and vegetables

- higher nutrient intakes

- lower intakes of soft drinks and fried food

- lower saturated fat intakes as a proportion of their total energy intake

Main meal basics

Choose a food or foods from each group – carbs, protein and fruit and vegetables.

1. **Start** with a low GI carb such as sweet potato, pasta, noodles, sweetcorn, beans, peas or lentils.
2. **Add** some protein such as lean meat or chicken, fish or seafood, eggs and pulses.
3. **Plus** plenty of vegetables and salad to help fill you up – remember our plate model (page 48). A large salad made with a variety of vegetables would be ideal. Round off the meal with fruit.

Alcohol

If you like to have a drink, that's OK – there might even be some health benefits. Both red and white wines contain powerful anti-oxidants, which may work to reduce heart disease risk. But go easy. While studies show some health benefits in those who drink one to two standard drinks a day, compared to none at all, there is a very steep increase in health risk from increased consumption. 100 ml/3½ fl oz (for women) to 200 ml/7 fl oz (for men) of wine per day is the maximum recommended by health authorities. Keep in mind that alcohol:

- is addictive
- can be fattening
- contributes to dehydration

Seven everyday low GI main meals

Peppered Steak with Sweet Potato Mash

1. **Carbohydrate**: sweet potato (allow 115 grams/4 oz per person)
2. **Protein**: fillet, rump or topside steak (allow 150 grams/ 5½ oz per person)
3. **Vegetables**: mushrooms, green beans, salad vegetables including tomato

Sprinkle steak with pepper seasoning and barbecue or pan-fry. Serve with steamed sweet potato mashed with skimmed milk, sliced mushrooms cooked in a little olive oil, steamed green beans and a crisp salad tossed in a vinaigrette dressing.

Lamb and Vegetables

1. **Carbohydrate**: canned or baby new potatoes (allow 2–3 per person), sweetcorn on the cob (allow 1 small cob per person)
2. **Protein**: trimmed lamb loin chops or cutlets (allow 200 grams/7 oz per person) or lean lamb fillet (allow 150 grams/5½ oz per person)
3. **Vegetables**: carrot, broccoli (allow 100 grams/3½ oz per person)

For extra flavour, coat the meat with a spice blend such as chermoula or garlic and rosemary and allow to 'dry marinate' for about 20 minutes. Barbecue or grill lamb (trim off the fat if you are cooking chops). Serve with steamed vegetables – baby new potatoes, corn cob, sliced carrots and broccoli florets – and your favourite condiments.

Thai-style Kebabs

1. **Carbohydrate**: basmati rice
2. **Protein**: chicken, beef, firm white-fleshed fish, or tofu (allow 500 grams/ 1 lb 2 oz for 4 kebabs)
3. **Vegetables**: courgette, onion, mushrooms (add extra vegetables such as red pepper if you like)

Prepare a marinade using the following ingredients: juice and grated rind of 2 limes, 1 teaspoon of crushed garlic, 1 tablespoon of grated ginger, 2 teaspoons of chopped chilli, 1 tablespoon of chopped lemongrass and 1 tablespoon of chopped coriander.

Marinate diced chicken, beef, firm fish or tofu, 2 courgettes sliced into rounds, 1 onion quartered and layers separated and 8 mushrooms, halved, or quartered if they are large, for at least 20 minutes, longer if you have the time. Thread the different ingredients alternately on skewers, brush with a little oil and barbecue or grill under a preheated grill for about 10 minutes, turning regularly and basting with the marinade. Serve with basmati rice and lime wedges.

Honey and Mustard Pork

1. **Carbohydrate**: baby new potatoes (allow 2–3 per person), or sweet potato (allow 115 grams /4 oz per person)
2. **Protein**: pork cutlets (allow 200 grams (7 oz) per person)
3. **Vegetables**: red pepper, broccoli

Prepare a marinade with the following: 1 tablespoon of olive oil, 1 tablespoon of seeded mustard, 2 teaspoons of honey, 2 tablespoons of lemon juice and freshly ground black pepper. Trim the fat off the pork cutlets, marinate for an hour then pan-fry for about 5 minutes on each side. Cut the peppers into strips lengthwise and stir-fry in the remaining marinade. Serve with steamed broccoli florets and potato or sweet potato, spooning the juices over the meat. Serve with additional mustard or apple sauce.

Spicy Fish with Rice and Vegetables

1. **Carbohydrate**: basmati rice
2. **Protein**: firm white fish fillets (allow 150 grams (5½ oz) per person)
3. **Vegetables**: frozen vegetable combination (peas, carrots, beans, sweetcorn, etc.)

Brush firm white fish fillets with your favourite curry paste blended with some lemon juice. Pan-fry and serve with basmati rice and steamed vegetables.

Spaghetti with Tomato Salsa and Feta

1. **Carbohydrate**: spaghetti (or your favourite pasta shapes)
2. **Protein**: feta cheese
3. **Vegetables**: tomato, onion, basil, olives, salad vegetables

To make enough salsa for 4 people, chop 4 tomatoes, ½ red onion, a handful of basil leaves and 75 grams (2½ oz) of pitted kalamata olives and combine in a bowl. Toss cooked spaghetti in a little olive oil and top with the tomato salsa and 150 grams (5½ oz) of crumbled feta. Serve with a crispy green salad.

Red Lentil and Vegetable Curry

1. Carbohydrate: split red lentils, basmati rice
2. Protein: lentils, yoghurt
3. Vegetables: onion, pumpkin, carrots, vegetable stock, spinach, coriander

Cook 1 finely chopped onion in a little oil in a large frying pan until soft and golden. Add 2 tablespoons of curry paste, 400 grams (14 oz) of diced pumpkin, 2 diced carrots and 125 grams (4½ oz) of split red lentils. Stir in 500 ml (17 fl oz) of vegetable stock and simmer, uncovered, until just cooked. Stir in the leaves from a bunch of spinach and simmer gently just until they wilt. Serve over steamed basmati rice with natural yoghurt, topped with finely chopped fresh coriander. Serves 4 people.

DESSERTS FOR
SWEET FINISHES

The idea of dessert puts a smile on everyone's face but so often we keep sweet treats for special occasions. Well, you don't need to worry with these recipe ideas – they are easy, everyday fare made with just a few ingredients in a matter of minutes. Finishing your meal with something sweet can help signal satiety/satisfaction to the brain's appetite centre, and stop you hunting around the kitchen afterwards. They're also a great source of fruit and calcium- and protein-rich dairy foods.

Seven everyday low GI desserts

Caramelised Apples

Cut 4 apples into quarters, remove the core and seeds and slice thinly. Cook in 1 tablespoon margarine for 4–5 minutes, or until golden. Reduce the heat and add 2 tablespoons brown sugar, stirring until it dissolves. Increase the heat and add 150 ml (5 fl oz) light evaporated milk and stir to combine and heat through. Serve the apples with the sauce and a dollop of low fat natural yoghurt.

Honey Banana Cups

Slice a large banana and halve 2 fresh passionfruit. Divide half a 200 gram (7 oz) pot of low fat honey-flavoured yoghurt between 2 small cups or glasses. Top with half the banana and one of the passionfruit. Top with the rest of the yoghurt and remaining banana, finishing with the passionfruit. Serve with a coconut macaroon alongside.

Health tip:

Low fat dairy products generally contain more calcium, phosphorus, potassium and magnesium than their full fat counterparts. So do your heart and your health a favour and eat lots of low fat dairy.

Strawberries with Honey Yoghurt

Toss 2 punnets of washed, hulled strawberries with 2 table-spoons of caster sugar in a frying pan for 5 minutes. Serve with low fat natural yoghurt combined with 1–2 table-spoons of honey, to taste.

Peaches with Cinnamon Ricotta

Beat 300 grams (10½ oz) of low fat ricotta cheese with 2 tablespoons of icing sugar, ½ teaspoon of cinnamon and ½ teaspoon of vanilla essence. Divide dollops of the mixture between 4 side plates and add a halved fresh peach (or any other fruit) and 2 almond wafers.

Banana Split

Cut 4 bananas in half lengthways and place in dessert bowls. Add 2 scoops of low fat ice-cream and top with the pulp of ½ passionfruit.

Summer Fruit Salsa

Dice a large mango, a handful of strawberries and a peeled orange into 1 cm (½ inch) pieces. Mix with fresh passion-fruit pulp and serve with low fat ice-cream or frozen yoghurt.

Fruit Toast

Toast thick slices of continental fruit loaf and spread with light cream cheese or ricotta sweetened with a teaspoonful of caster sugar and a few drops of vanilla essence. Top with fresh fruit: sliced banana, peach or strawberries, or whole fresh blueberries or raspberries. Sprinkle with icing sugar to serve.

Sugar

Many people pride themselves on not keeping sugar in their larder, yet have a bottle of fruit juice in the fridge. Sure, fruit juice does provide vitamin C and other phytonutrients but it also contains about five teaspoons of sugar per glass, the same as soft drink.

Sugar can be a concentrated source of calories, with few nutrients, but no more so than a bottle of oil or alcoholic spirits or a block of butter. It isn't advisable to consume sugar to excess but you can use it in moderation without adversely affecting your health.

TIME FOR A SNACK

Most people feel like eating every three to four hours. Eating frequently can help you avoid becoming too hungry and lessen the chance of overeating when meal times come around. Depending on what you choose, snacks can also make a valuable contribution to your vitamin and mineral intake.

Quick snacks you can make anytime

- fresh fruit salad
- a handful of fresh or frozen grapes

- vegetable sticks with hummous or yoghurt-based dip: cut fresh celery, cucumber, carrots, red peppers and courgettes
- low fat natural yoghurt with fresh fruit
- a smoothie made with fruit and skimmed milk and yoghurt
- a scoop (just one!) of low fat ice-cream
- hummous with pitta bread
- a bowl of cereal with low fat milk
- a slice of fruit or raisin toast
- an apple muffin
- 2 oat biscuits with a slice of cheese and an apple
- wholewheat breakfast biscuits with milk (Note: eating sweetened cereals dry is hazardous for teeth – always add milk.)

How to make pitta chips

Open out Lebanese bread, spread lightly with bottled sweet chilli sauce and grill until just crisp.

Portable pack-and-go snacks

- a juicy orange
- a small banana
- a large peach or pear
- single-serve pear or peach snack pack in natural juice
- a handful of dried fruit and nut mix
- a handful of dried apricots, apple rings, sultanas or raisins
- a pot of low fat yoghurt or a dairy dessert
- low fat cheese or cheese sticks
- popcorn
- 4 squares (25–30 grams/about 1 oz) of chocolate (very occasionally for a treat)

Hot snacks for cold days

- corn on the cob
- a mug of vegetable soup with toast or crackers
- toasted sandwich on low GI bread

- small can of baked beans
- small serving of instant noodles with vegetables
- toasted fruit loaf lightly spread with margarine or low fat ricotta
- low GI toast fingers lightly spread with Nutella®, peanut butter, honey, fruit spread or Marmite®

Nibbles

- a small handful of unsalted, roasted nuts
- a small handful of dried fruit and nut mix
- carrot, celery and other vegetable sticks
- fruit platter – berries, orange segments, dried fruit, nuts, etc.
- marinated vegetable platter (use paper towels to soak up some of the oil before arranging the platter) with pitta bread

Drinks

- a small glass of fruit juice (150 ml/5 fl oz)
- low fat milk or calcium-enriched soya milk
- low fat flavoured milk
- warm flavoured milk drink (Milo®, Horlicks®, Ovaltine® etc.)
- a low fat smoothie
- café latte or cappuccino with semi-skimmed milk

 ## Health tip:

Make a delicious low fat milkshake by combining a cup of low fat milk with a tablespoon of skimmed milk powder, 2 tablespoons of low fat vanilla yoghurt and a tablespoon of ice-cream topping. Blend until frothy.

WHAT TO DRINK?

Water

It's calorie-free and cheap – surely two good reasons for drinking water. However, it isn't necessary to drink eight glasses a day. Food contributes at least one-third of our daily fluid requirement, so we need five to seven cups of fluid to make up the remainder. Aim to make at least two or three of these water.

Fruit juice

It's widely considered a healthy drink, but if your diet includes fruit and vegetables, fruit juice really isn't necessary. If you like to include it, one glass (150 ml/5 fl oz) a day is enough, and think of it as a (low fibre) serving of fruit.

Tea

Drinking a cup of tea often provides the opportunity to take time out and relax – there is a benefit in this. Tea has also been recognised recently as a valuable source of anti-oxidants which may protect against several forms of cancer, cardiovascular disease, kidney stones, bacterial infection and dental cavities. A maximum of two to three cups of tea a day is recommended.

Coffee

Did you know that 80 per cent of the world's population consumes caffeine daily? For most people, no more than two cups of coffee a day is recommended, but if you are pregnant, caffeine sensitive or have high blood pressure it is probably best to cut down to one cup per day. Both tea and coffee are a major source of anti-oxidants in the diet, simply because they are so widely and frequently consumed.

> Energy drinks available in the UK that have been GI tested so far are Gatorade®, Isostar® and Lucozade®, and all have a high GI. This means they are a rapidly available source of glucose and makes them better suited to fluid replacement after strenuous exercise. For the recreational couch potato they may be just adding extra calories.

Three tips for making the switch

1. Start with something easy.

2. Do it gradually.

3. Don't expect 100 per cent.

Milk

Milk is a valuable source of nutrients for adults and children but, being a liquid, it is easily overconsumed. Think of it as food in a liquid form. Recommended intakes vary for different ages, but for normal, healthy, non-pregnant adults, around 300–450 ml (10½–16 fl oz) of semi-skimmed milk a day is suitable.

LIVING EVERYDAY LOW GI EATING

Five typical menus

Wondering if you can really make this low GI diet work for you? Here's how some of our readers have changed to everyday low GI eating.

Barbara, 65, small eater

'When I gave up work to become a full-time home-maker I found I piled on the weight – and I wasn't happy about that at all! I keep myself busy looking after the house, my husband and my three young grandchildren several times a week. To get myself back into shape, I go for a brisk walk for at least 20 minutes, sometimes 40 minutes, in the morning, as often as I can. I've been eating low GI food for a year now and I'm used to it. That's just the way I (and my husband) eat now. I've lost 10 kilograms (22 lb) so far – down to 82 kilograms (12 stone 9 lb), but I'd like to lose a lot more!'

Breakfast

- small cranberry juice
- 30 grams (1 oz) Guardian® with 125 ml (4 fl oz) semi-skimmed milk
- white tea with 1 sugar

Mid-morning

- low fat yoghurt
- 1 fresh apricot

Lunch

- cheese and tomato sandwich on multigrain bread (with light margarine)
- white tea

Mid-afternoon

- 1 peach

Dinner

- grilled trout fillet
- 2 small jacket potatoes
- mixed salad
- low fat ice-cream in cone

After-dinner snack

- small bunch grapes
- 6 almonds

Harry, 55, medium eater

'I am on the road as a sales rep. I'd like to lose weight to look better – I actually need to lose about 20 kilograms (3 stone). Because my job is quite sedentary – I spend so much time sitting at a desk or behind the wheel of a car – I make the effort to walk for half an hour most weekday mornings. On the weekend I'll do a longer walk for an hour or so. So far I have lost 8 kilograms (18 lb). I eat out most lunchtimes and I'm now a three-meals-a-day person and I'll eat in between if I get hungry. It was a big change for me to start eating breakfast.'

Breakfast

- 2 slices multigrain toast spread with light margarine plus 2 slices of low fat processed cheese and half a tomato
- 1 banana

Mid-morning

- skinny cappuccino

Lunch

- 1 bowl miso soup
- teppanyaki chicken
- salad
- 200 grams (7 oz) cooked Japanese sushi rice

Dinner

- 200 grams (7 oz) cooked spaghetti
- 200 grams (7 oz) meat and tomato sauce
- 1 dessert bowl green salad
- 1 banana
- 1 fresh peach
- 100 grams (3½ oz) fat-free yoghurt
- glass of chardonnay

Fiona, 38, medium eater

'I have a more-than-fulltime, stressful job and work long hours. I have little time for planned exercise, so rely on 'incidental exercise' around the office or shopping, etc. I am not trying to lose weight – but I don't want to gain any! So I am careful with my diet and fussy about the food I eat. I take my lunch to work – it saves time and I know I am eating healthily!'

Breakfast

- small freshly squeezed orange juice
- 50 grams (1¾ oz) muesli with natural yoghurt
- a nectarine
- tea with low fat milk

Mid-morning

- nut bar
- tea with low fat milk

Lunch

- 2–3 slices grain bread, no butter
- mixed salad
- 100 gram (3½ oz) can tuna or salmon
- salad dressing
- grapes

Mid-afternoon

- white coffee
- low fat fruit yoghurt
- an apple

Did you know?

Eating just half a cup of broccoli each week is enough to boost your health. Imagine what more could do!

Dinner

- 150 grams (5½ oz) chicken strips
- 200 grams (7 oz) stir-fried noodles
- 400 grams (14 oz) stir-fried vegetables

After-dinner snack

- 2 scoops of low fat ice-cream or a choc-chip biscuit

David, 50, bigger eater

'I work fulltime as a warehouse manager, which I guess could be classified as 'light activity' – my job certainly gives me a good level of incidental activity. I socialise a fair bit and go square dancing twice a week. I have lost 10 kilograms (22 lb) and am now maintaining stable weight. I wouldn't really say I'm on a diet. We just eat well, we made a few changes to our bread and I eat more fruit than I used to.'

Breakfast

- 30 grams (1 oz) Special K® with 10 grams (⅓ oz) All-Bran® with 200 ml (7 fl oz) semi-skimmed milk
- ½ sliced banana

Mid-morning

- an apple and a banana

Lunch

- 4 slices grainy bread
- low fat cheese and ham
- pickles, tomato, lettuce
- diet drink

Mid-afternoon

- 3–4 oatmeal cookies or home-made muesli slice
- white coffee

Dinner

- lean steak
- 2 new potatoes, plus a chunk of sweet potato
- mini corn cob
- broccoli, carrot, pumpkin, beans

Dessert

- canned fruit and 125 ml (4 fl oz) low fat custard

Did you know?

An 85-gram (3 oz) packet of instant noodles supplies as many calories as five slices of bread. Low GI they may be, but low calorie they definitely are not.

Vicki, 29, medium eater

'I am a vegetarian but I do eat dairy foods. I work full-time in an office. I catch a train to work so I accumulate about 30 minutes of walking each day. On the weekends I do lots of outdoors things – go to the beach, swim, walks. Although I don't need to watch my weight, I am aware that I need to get plenty of iron from my diet. Eating low GI foods, I just feel better and have more energy to do things. It's the ideal way of eating to me!'

Breakfast

- 30 grams (1 oz) Ultra-Bran Soy and Linseed cereal with 2 tablespoons low fat plain yoghurt, skimmed milk and a small handful of raisins
- skim latte (decaf!)

Mid-morning

- 1 nectarine
- herbal tea

Lunch

- Avocado sushi roll, tofu sushi roll

Mid-afternoon

- 1 apple and a small handful of cashews
- tea with milk

Dinner

- 2 tortillas with red kidney bean and lentil chilli sauce with light sour cream, grated cheese and lettuce
- green side salad with vinaigrette

CLUED IN ON EATING OUT?

Quite often it's the high-calorie (kilojoule) foods you unknowingly choose from the menu that tip your healthy eating plans out of balance. If you eat out more than once a week, it's worth thinking about what you're actually eating. Check out your knowledge with this quick quiz.

Which of these has the lowest fat content?

a) combination Chinese meal with fried rice/lemon chicken/sweet and sour pork
b) lasagne with meat
c) Japanese bento box including beef with rice, sushi and salad
d) fish and chips, including battered fish

Which is the lowest calorie option when you catch up for coffee?

a) skimmed-milk hot chocolate
b) cappuccino
c) skimmed-milk latte

Which drink is less fattening?

a) Bacardi Breezer

b) Corona beer

c) glass of wine

Which is the healthiest fast-food snack?

a) 2 slices of super-supreme pizza

b) roast chicken Subway® sub with cheese

c) chicken burger

Which light meal is a low GI choice?

a) grilled chicken, avocado, pepper and cheese toasted Turkish bread sandwich

b) wedges with sour cream and sweet chilli sauce

c) fettuccine Napolitana

Which makes the healthiest café snack?

a) chunky raisin toast and butter

b) low fat banana smoothie

c) carrot cake

The secrets revealed

Which of these has the lowest fat content?

The meat lasagne is the lowest fat option here with an average serving containing only 16 grams of fat. Next is the Japanese Bento Box at 33 grams; fish and chips at 35; and a massive 40 grams in the Chinese meal.

Which is the lowest calorie option when you catch up for coffee?

The skimmed milk latte is the winner here in terms of calories (335 kJ/80 Kcal, 0.5 grams fat) and has the added bonus of extra calcium. Although the hot chocolate is made with skimmed milk it has twice the calories (670 kJ/160 Kcal) and eight times the fat. The cappuccino is in between at 375 kJ/90 Kcal and 5 grams of fat.

Which drink is less fattening?

Depending on your knowledge of alcoholic beverages, you might have guessed that the glass of wine is least fattening, containing the lowest number of calories. It's closely followed by the beer at 545 kJ/130 Kcal and the 'alcopop' Bacardi Breezer tops the list at 880 kJ/210 Kcal per serve. That's as much as three slices of bread!

Which is the healthiest fast-food snack?

Subway® fast food can be a lower calorie snack, depending on your toppings, but it whacks a pretty high glycaemic load on your plate with even the standard 'sub' which contains 44 grams of carbohydrate, and bread which is probably high GI (it hasn't been tested). None of the other options here are any better in the GI stakes and are all higher in calories.

Which light meal is a low GI choice?

Pasta has a low GI, so the fettuccine is the best option. Potato and refined flour in the other choices make them high GI. All of these options will have a high GL because of their large carbohydrate content, so team the pasta with salad and pass on the garlic bread!

Which makes the healthiest café snack?

Sustaining, nutritious and delicious – how could you go past a banana smoothie for a premium low GI snack? The raisin toast also has a low GI, but is best with the butter served separately so you control the amount.

MAKING THE RIGHT CHOICES WHEN EATING OUT

Fast-food outlets

Burgers and French fries are a bad idea – quickly eaten, high in saturated fat and rapidly absorbed high GI carbs that fill you with calories that don't last long. Some fast-food chains are introducing healthier choices but read the fine print. Look out for lean protein, low GI carbs, good fats and lots of vegetables.

You can choose:

- **marinated and barbecued chicken**, rather than fried
- **salads** such as coleslaw or garden salad; eat the salad first
- **corn on the cob** as a healthy side order
- **individual menu items** rather than meal deals, and never upsize

Lunch bars

Steer clear of places displaying lots of deep-fried fare and head towards fresh food bars offering fruit and vegetables. Tubs of garden or Greek salad finished with fruit and yoghurt make a healthy, low GI choice.

With sandwiches and melts, choose the fillings carefully. Including cheese can make the fat exceed 20 grams (¾ oz) per sandwich (that's as much as chips!).

Make sure you include some vegetables or salad in or alongside the sandwich.

You can choose:

- **mixed grain** bread rather than white
- **salad** fillings for sandwiches or as a side order instead of chips

- **pasta** dishes with both vegetables and meat
- **Lebanese kebabs** with tabbouleh and hummous
- **grilled fish** rather than fried
- **vegetarian pizza**
- **gourmet wraps**

In cafés

Whether it's a quick snack or a main meal, catching up with a friend for coffee doesn't have to tip your diet off balance. Pass on breads, but if you really must, something like a dense Italian bread is better than a garlic or herb bread.

Whatever you order, specify: 'no French fries – extra salad instead' so temptation does not confront you. If you want something sweet try a skimmed iced chocolate or a single little biscuit or slice.

You can choose:

- **semi-skimmed** or **skimmed milk coffee** rather than full cream milk
- **sourdough** or **wholegrain bread** instead of white or wholemeal
- **bruschetta** with tomatoes, onions, olive oil and basil on a dense Italian bread rather than buttery herb or garlic bread
- **salad** as a main or side order, with the dressing served separately so you control the amount
- **char-grilled steak** or **chicken breast** rather than fried or crumbed
- **vegetable-topped pizza** – such as pepper, onion, mushroom, artichoke, aubergine
- **lean meat pizza** – such as ham, fresh seafood or sliced chicken breast
- **pasta** with sauces such as marinara; Bolognese; Napolitana; arrabiata (tomato with olives, roasted pepper

and chilli); and piccolo (aubergine, roasted pepper and artichoke)

- **seafood** such as marinated calamari, grilled with chilli and lemon or steamed mussels with a tomato sauce
- **water, mineral water** or **freshly squeezed fruit and vegetable** juices rather than soft drinks

Asian meals

Asian meals including Chinese, Thai, Indian and Japanese offer a great variety of foods, making it possible to select a healthy meal with some careful choices.

Keeping in line with the 1, 2, 3 steps to a balanced meal, seek out a low GI carb such as basmati rice, dhal, sushi or noodles. Chinese and Thai rice will traditionally be jasmine and although high GI, a small serve of steamed rice is better for you than fried rice or noodles.

Next add some protein – marinated tofu, stir-fried seafood, Tandoori chicken, fish tikka or a braised dish with vegetables. Be cautious with pork and duck, for which fattier cuts are often used; and avoid Thai curries and dishes made with coconut milk because it's high in saturated fat.

And don't forget, the third dish to order is stir-fried vegetables!

You can choose:

- **steamed dumplings, dim sum** or **fresh spring rolls** rather than fried entrees
- **clear soups** to fill you up, rather than high fat laksa
- **noodles** in soups rather than fried in dishes such as pad Thai
- **noodle and vegetable stir-fries** – if you ask for extra vegetables you may find that the one dish feeds two
- **seafood** braised in a sauce with vegetables
- **tofu (bean curd), chicken, beef, lamb** or **pork fillet** braised with nuts, vegetables, black bean or other sauces

- **salads** such as Thai salads
- **smaller serves of rice**
- **vegetable dishes** such as stir-fried vegetables, vegetable curry, dhal, channa (a delicious chickpea curry) and side orders such as pickles, cucumber and yoghurt, tomato and onion
- **Japanese dishes** such as sushi, teriyaki, sashimi, salmon steak or tuna, teppanyaki (which is char-grilled) in preference to tempura, which is deep-fried

Airlines and airports

Airports are notoriously bad places to eat – fast-food chains, a limited range, pre-made sandwiches, sad-looking cakes, a lack of fresh fruit and vegetables – and it's expensive!

In airline lounges you will do better, although, again, the range is limited. Fresh fruit is always on offer and usually some sort of vegetables either as salad or soup. The bread is usually the super-high GI white French type and with crackers as the only other option, you would do better to rely on fruit, fruit juices, yoghurt or a skimmed milk coffee for your carbs.

In-flight, unless you have the privilege of a sky chef, meals are fairly standard fare, including a salad and fruit if you're lucky. Many airlines offer special diets with advance bookings and although there's no guarantee it meets your nutritional criteria, it may give you healthier choices compared to what everyone else is having.

Travelling domestic economy these days, it's probably best to eat before you leave, take your own snacks with you and decline the in-flight snack (you really will be better off without that mini chocolate bar, biscuit, cake or muffin, and on some airlines you have to pay for it).

You can choose to eat:

- **fresh fruit, soup** and **salad items** in airline lounges rather than white bread, cheese, cakes and salami
- **small meals** in-flight, rather than eating everything put in front of you
- **water** to drink, wherever you are
- **dried fruit, nut bars, bananas** or **apples** that you have taken along yourself

WHAT TO PUT IN THE SHOPPING TROLLEY

The perfect place to get started on healthy low GI eating is the supermarket, whether you are pushing a trolley up and down the aisles, or shopping online. This is where we make those hurried or impulsive decisions that have a big impact. If you see chocolate on sale, do you stock up or keep walking? One little decision – what a big impact.

Make a list

Spend a little time each day, or weekly if it suits, planning what to eat when. It makes life simpler. Meal planning is just writing down what you intend to eat for the main meals of the week, then checking your fridge and pantry for ingredients available and noting what you need to purchase. We've included more ideas on meal planning in the menu section on pages 49–64. So study the GI tables, look at the meal ideas in this book and browse through some recipes with a notepad handy.

The shopping list on pages 87–90 is just to get you started. Bear in mind that it doesn't contain all low GI foods, and individual choices will be dictated by your tastes and budget. Make a photocopy and take it with you to the shops if you like, or just use it for ideas. For more tips on what to pop in the trolley and stock in your pantry, check out Part 3: The Top 100 Low GI Food Finder.

WHY IT'S IMPORTANT TO READ THE LABEL

Often we're asked questions like: 'What should I look for on the label?' and 'Can I believe what it says?'

Reading the fine print

Remember, the GI alone doesn't identify a healthy food. If you like to keep some numbers in your head when you're shopping, then the following details are for you. Keep in mind that they are a general guide and shouldn't be used definitively to exclude or include foods in your diet.

Health tip:

Remember, if you don't buy it, you can't eat it.

Energy – This is a measure of how many kilojoules (kJ) or calories (Kcal) we get from a food. For a healthy diet we need to eat more foods with a low energy density and combine them with smaller amounts of higher energy foods. To assess the energy density of a packaged food, look at the kJ or Kcal per 100 grams. A low energy density is less than 500 kJ per 100 grams or 120 Kcals per 100 grams.

Fat – Seek low saturated fat content, ideally less than 20 per cent of the total fat. For example, if the total fat content is 10 grams, you want saturated fat to be less than 2 grams. A food can be labelled as being low fat only if it contains less than 1.5 grams of saturated fat per 100 grams/100 ml and the saturated fat provides less than 10 per cent of the total energy of the product.

Carbohydrate – This is the starch plus any naturally occurring and added sugars in the food. There's no need to look at the sugar figure separately since it's the total carbohydrate that affects your blood glucose level. You could use the total carbohydrate figure if you were monitoring your carbohydrate intake and to calculate the GL of the serving. The GL = grams of total carbohydrate x GI/100.

Sample Nutritional Information

Typical values per 100 grams

Energy	245kJ/58 Kcal
Protein	4.6 g
Carbohydrate	7.2 g
of which sugars	6.5 g
Fat	1.2 g
of which saturates	0.2 g
Fibre	0.2 g
Sodium	0.1 g

For more information on food labelling go to **www.eatwell.gov.uk/foodlabels**

Can I believe what it says?

Consumers are increasingly interested in what is in the food they eat. That's where the Food Standards Agency (FSA) comes in. This independent food safety watchdog was set up by an act of parliament to provide consumers and government with advice and information on nutrition and diet, and on food safety from farm to fork. It also protects consumers through effective monitoring and enforcement of regulations. For more information visit: www.food.gov.uk or www.eatwell.gov.uk

Fibre – Most of us don't eat enough fibre in our diet (the average intake for adults in the UK is around 12 grams a day – 6 grams short of the recommended 18 grams a day). So seek out foods that are high in fibre. Foods and food products that contain 6 grams of fibre per 100 grams (or 100 ml) may be labelled as being a 'high fibre' food.

Sodium – This is a measure of the nasty part of salt in our food. Our bodies need some salt but many people consume much more salt than the 6 grams a day they need. Canned, convenience and ready-to-eat foods in particular tend to be high in sodium. When shopping, check the nutrition label for the sodium content. If a food contains between 0.1 grams and 0.5 grams of sodium per 100 grams, this could be considered a moderate amount. A small amount would be less than 0.1 grams of sodium per 100 grams of the food. Sometimes sodium is listed in milligrams (mg). There are 1000 mg in 1 gram, so 600 mg = 0.6 grams and 1200 mg = 1.2 grams. For more information on sodium and salt go to www.salt.gov.uk

Health tip:

Seventy-five per cent of most people's salt intake comes from the supermarket (in processed foods and ready-to-eat meals) and from takeaways. What can you do to cut down?

- Check the labels for sodium content.
- Never add salt to your food.
- Minimise the frequency with which you eat salty foods.

How do you know if it's low, medium or high GI?

When it comes to the supermarket shelves, it's getting easier to identify foods that have been GI tested by the use of special GI symbols. Unfortunately, however, not all claims are reliable. Why? Well, the GI rating of a food must be tested physiologically and only a few centres around the world currently provide such a testing service. In fact the GI is defined by its internationally standardised method of testing in human subjects (we call this in vivo testing). You may hear about in vitro (test tube) methods, but these are simple short cuts, which may be useful for food manufacturers developing new products, but may not reflect the true GI of a food.

The GI Symbol Program

This international symbol is a guarantee that the product meets the Sydney University GI Research Service (SUGiRS) program's strict nutritional criteria. Whether high, medium or low GI, you can be assured that these foods are healthier choices within their food group. A number of leading food manufacturers in Australia have had their products GI tested by SUGiRS, an international program established by the University of Sydney, Diabetes Australia and the Juvenile Diabetes Research Foundation.

Some supermarket chains in the UK are glycaemic index testing products and labelling them 'Low GI' or 'Medium GI'.

Sainsbury's

Sainsbury's launched low and medium GI labelling progressively across a range of products that meet strict nutritional criteria and that were tested by the Hammersmith Food Research Unit at Hammersmith Hospital.

Tesco

Tesco launched GI labelling across a range of products that were tested by Oxford Brookes University. Products are labelled 'Low Gi' or 'Medium Gi'.

EVERYDAY LOW GI SHOPPING

Having the staples on hand

Our shopping list will help you stock the larder and refrigerator with the staples you require to turn out a meal in minutes. It includes everything you'll need for the low GI meal ideas in the food finder.

To make your own shopping list, use the same headings. They will take you to the appropriate aisles of the supermarket or to the shops you usually favour.

We've included convenience foods such as canned beans, bagged salads, bottled sauces and pastes, canned fruits and chopped vegetables (fresh and frozen) in the list. There's no need to feel guilty about using these items. Remember, this book is about making eating a healthy, low GI diet as easy as possible and although some convenience items such as frozen vegetables or canned beans may be a little more expensive, the time savings and health benefits can outweigh the costs.

If you want to know more about some of the foods on the shopping list, check the food finder in Part 3. We have included lots of meal ideas and even some recipes in this section.

 Health tip:

We need to eat foods with fibre for bowel health and to keep regular. In fact we need about 18 grams of fibre a day (most of us fall short of that – about 6 grams short). It's easy to increase your intake. Just make sure your shopping list includes high fibre breakfast cereals and porridge oats, wholegrain or granary breads, fresh fruit and vegetables and canned (or dried) beans, peas and lentils. You'll find plenty of ideas for using these low GI high fibre foods in our Top 100 Food Finder.

The bakery

Fruit loaf

Low GI bread
  Granary or wholegrain
  Sourdough

English-style muffins

Pitta bread

The refrigerated cabinet

Milk
  Semi-skimmed
  Skimmed
  Low fat flavoured
Margarine
Cheese
  Reduced fat grated
  cheese
  Parmesan cheese
  Reduced fat ricotta
  or cottage cheese
  Reduced fat cheese
  slices
Yoghurt
  Low fat plain/natural
  Low fat fruit or vanilla
  flavoured
  Low fat drinking
  yoghurt

Soya alternatives
  Low fat calcium-enriched
  soya milk
  Soya yoghurt
Dairy desserts
  Crème fraîche desserts
  Custard
Fruit juice
  Apple juice
  Orange juice
  Grapefruit juice
  Cranberry juice
Fresh noodles
Fresh pasta
  Ravioli
  Tortellini
Tofu
Sushi
Dips such as hummous

Your everyday checkout choice

To cut back the fat, choose:

- lean cuts of meat and skinless chicken

- low fat dairy and soya milk products

- vegetable oils and cooking sprays

- 'lite' spreads and dressings

- tomato and pepper sauces and salsas to serve with pasta

Health tip:

If they have been stored and cooked carefully, frozen vegetables can provide similar levels of nutrients to those of fresh vegetables, sometimes even more.

The freezer

Ice-cream
  Reduced or low fat
  vanilla or flavoured
  Frozen yoghurt
Frozen fruit desserts
or gelato
Frozen vegetables
  Peas

Beans
Corn
Spinach
Mixed vegetables
Stir-fry mix
Broccoli
Cauliflower

> **Your everyday checkout choice**
>
> To fill up with fibre choose a cereal containing at least 9 grams of fibre per 100 grams.

Fresh fruit and vegetables

Basics
  Sweet potato
  Yam
  Sweetcorn
  Lemons or limes
  Onions
  Carrots
  Garlic
  Ginger
  Chillies
Leafy green and other
seasonal vegetables
  Spinach or silverbeet
  Cabbage
  Broccoli
  Cauliflower
  Asparagus
  Asian greens such
  as bok choi
  Leeks
  Fennel
  Mangetout

Beans and peas
Courgette or marrow
Brussel sprouts
Aubergine
Mushrooms
Salad vegetables, depending
on season
  Lettuce (choose a variety)
  Rocket
  Tomato
  Cucumber
  Pepper
  Spring onions
  Celery
  Bagged mixed salad
  greens
  Sprouts – mung bean,
  mangetout, alfalfa etc.
  Avocado
  Fresh herbs, depending
  on season
  Parsley

> **Your everyday checkout choice**
>
> To bone up on calcium choose low fat dairy products.

Basil

Mint

Chives

Coriander

Fresh fruit, depending

on season

　Apples

　Oranges

Pears

Grapes

Grapefruit

Peaches

Apricots

Strawberries and other

berries

Mango

General groceries

Eggs

Beverages

　Tea

　Coffee

　Flavoured milk

　powders such as

　Milo®, Horlicks®

　or Ovaltine®

Herbs, spices, condiments

and sauces

　Tube or jar of minced

　ginger, garlic, chilli

　Mustard

　Creamed horseradish

　Tomato sauce

　Asian sauces

　Soy sauce

　Bottled pasta sauce

　Jar of curry paste

Deli items or pre-packed jars

　Sundried tomatoes

　Olives

Spreads

　Pure floral honey

　Apricot jam

Nutella®

Peanut butter

Marmite®

Oils and vinegars

　Rapeseed or olive oil

　cooking spray

　Olive oil

　Rapeseed or vegetable oil

　Balsamic vinegar

　White wine vinegar

Breakfast cereals

　Traditional rolled oats

　Natural muesli

　Low GI packaged

　breakfast cereal

Cereals and wholegrains

　Pasta

　Noodles, rice, buckwheat

　Rice – basmati or

　Japanese sushi rice

　such as Koshihikari

　Couscous

　Bulghur/cracked wheat

　Pearl barley

　Oat biscuits

Did you know?

Highly processed breakfast cereals have high GI values, not because they're high in sugar but because they're high in refined starch.

Your everyday checkout choice

To increase iron intake choose lean red meat.

Dried pulses
  Beans – keep a variety in the cupboard including cannellini, borlotti, lima, kidney, soya, pinto etc.
  Chickpeas
  Lentils
  Split peas
Canned foods, including pulses
  Baked beans
  Mexi-beans
  Chickpeas
  Lentils
  Beans – keep a variety in the cupboard including cannellini, butter, borlotti, lima, kidney, soya, pinto etc
  Four bean mix
  Corn kernels

Tomatoes, whole, crushed and tomato paste
Tomato soup
Tuna packed in spring water or oil
Salmon packed in water
Sardines
Canned fruit and single serve pots
  Pears
  Peaches
  Mixed fruit salad
Dried fruit and nuts
  Apricots
  Sultanas
  Raisins
  Prunes
  Apple rings
  Unsalted natural almonds, walnuts, cashews, etc.

Butcher/meat department

Lean ham
Lean beef for grills, barbecues and casseroles
Lean lamb fillets
Lean pork fillets
Lean minced beef

Chicken
  Skinless chicken breast or drumsticks
Fish
  Any type of fresh fish

Health tip:

Low iron levels can cause tiredness, physical weakness and increased sensitivity to cold. Lean red meat is a rich and highly bio-available source of iron, so aim to include it in your diet at least three times a week.

READY . . . SET . . . GO – MOVE IT & LOSE IT!

When we explained the basics of everyday low GI eating at the beginning of this section, we mentioned that one of the golden rules is to accumulate 60 minutes of physical activity every day, including incidental activity and planned exercise. This will help you control your weight for a whole host of reasons. To make a real difference to your health and energy levels, exercise has to be regular and some of it needs to be aerobic. But every little bit counts – and, best of all, any extra exercise you do is a step in the right direction.

> Remember, all you have to do is accumulate 60 minutes of physical activity every day.

Though some people can make a serious commitment to 30-plus minutes of planned exercise three or four times a week, most of us have a long list of excuses. We're too busy, too tired, too rushed, too stressed, too hot, too cold to go to the gym or take a walk or do a regular exercise routine. But there's good news. Research tells us that the calories we burn in our everyday activities are important too, and that any amount of movement is better than none at all.

Changing the habits of a lifetime isn't easy. We know how hard it can be to find time to fit everything into a day, especially if you are working and have a family. That's why we suggest you move it and lose it with our '1, 2, 3 one step at a time, in your own time' approach.

1. *Start* with extra incidental activity.
2. *Add* time to move more.
3. *Plus* planned exercise – it's worth it.

1. Start with extra incidental activity

> Think of extra incidental activity as an opportunity, not an inconvenience.

Incidental activity is the exercise we accumulate each day as part of our normal routines – putting out the rubbish, making the bed, doing chores, walking to the bus stop, popping out for a coffee and walking up a flight of stairs. If you make a conscious effort to increase the amount of this kind of activity in your day, it will eventually become second nature.

With just a little extra effort, here's how you can build more incidental physical activity into your life. You've probably heard these ideas before, so read this list as a timely reminder. It would be great if you could use just one of these ideas regularly.

- Use the stairs instead of taking the lift. Walk up them as quickly as you can. Try taking them two at a time – to strengthen your legs.
- Don't stand still on the escalator – walk up and down.
- Take the long way around whenever you can – popping down to the corner shop, getting a drink from the office water cooler, going to the bathroom.
- Make the time to walk your children to or from school.
- Catch up with a friend by meeting for a walk, rather than talking on the phone or over coffee.
- Get off your chair and talk to your colleagues rather than sending endless emails.
- Walk the dog instead of hitting tennis balls for him or her to chase and retrieve.
- Get rid of the leaf blower and rake the leaves or sweep the courtyard the old-fashioned way.

- Park the car at the opposite end of the carpark and walk to the cash machine, post office or dry cleaners.
- Walk to a restaurant (or park a good distance from it) to force yourself to take a walk after dinner.

Think of extra incidental activity as an opportunity not an inconvenience. The following table shows how 'spending' five minutes here and there every day can add up to potential fat 'savings' in the long term.

Take 5 minutes everyday to:	Potential savings in kilos of fat*	
	in 1 year	in 5 years
Take the stairs instead of the lift	3.7	18.5
Vacuum the living room	0.7	3.5
Walk 150 metres from the car to the office	0.7	3.5
Carry the groceries 150 metres to the car	0.9	4.5

* Figures based on a 70 kg (11 stone) person

2. Add time to move more

Exercise is more likely to be achieved when scheduled into your day, just like any other appointment. So think about your day, make a note in your diary and prioritise exercise. To reap the benefits, exercise doesn't have to be intense: exercise of moderate duration and intensity – including walking – is associated with reduced risk of disease. While brisk walking is best, even slow walkers benefit!

For most of us, walking fits the bill perfectly. It keeps us fit, it's cheap and convenient, it gets us out and about, and

If you do regular exercise you:

- will tend to have lower blood pressure
- will feel more energetic
- are less likely to have a heart attack or develop diabetes
- will reduce your insulin requirements if you have diabetes
- will find it easier to stop smoking
- will be better able to control your weight
- can increase levels of 'good' HDL cholesterol
- will sleep better

If you do regular exercise you:

- will have stronger bones and muscles

- are less likely to develop colon cancer

- will feel happier, more confident and relaxed

- can ease depression

it becomes even more important as we grow older. You can walk alone, or with friends. In fact, talking while you walk can have important emotional benefits: Not only do our bodies produce calming hormones while we walk, but the talk itself can be great therapy – and good for relationships in general. But don't hesitate to walk alone if you prefer, or with your dog – your pet will love you all the more for it. And you'll be able to take some time to think and relax.

How often? Try to walk every day. Ideally you should accumulate 30 minutes or more on most days of the week. The good news is, you can do it in two 15-minute sessions or six 5-minute sessions. It doesn't matter.

How hard? You should be able to talk comfortably while you walk. Find a level that suits you. If you feel sore at first, don't worry; your body will adapt and the soreness will decrease. Stretching for 2 minutes before and after your walk will help minimise aches and pains.

Getting started Before beginning a walking (or any exercise) program, see your doctor if you have:

- been inactive for some time
- a history of heart disease or chest pains
- diabetes
- high blood pressure

Or if you:

- smoke
- weigh more than you should

Health tip

For more information, step out and check out these walking programs:
www.whi.org.uk
www.ramblers.org.uk
www.healthierweight.co.uk
www.foodfitness.org.uk
www.everydaysport.com

How many steps will make a difference?

Go out and buy a cheap pedometer (step counter). Research has shown that every day we need to take about:

- ❑ 7500 steps to maintain weight
- ❑ 10 000 steps to lose weight
- ❑ 12 500 steps to prevent weight regain

For most of us this means taking a walk on top of our incidental activity. In the normal course of a day – just living and working – it is virtually impossible (unless you deliver the mail or walk other people's dogs for a living!) to achieve that 10 000 steps a day. The following table gives you an idea of how many steps are equivalent to 15 minutes of certain activities.

15 minutes of activity	Equivalent number of steps
Moderate sexual activity	500
Watering the garden	600
Vigorous sexual activity	750
Clearing and washing the dishes	900
Standing cooking at the barbecue	950
Standing while playing with kids	1100
Carpentry – general workshop	1200
Playing golf at the driving range	1200
Food shopping with a trolley	1400
General house cleaning	1400
Sweeping and raking	1600
Digging the garden	2000
Mowing the lawn with a hand mower	2350
Moving furniture	2350
Carrying bricks or using heavy tools	3150

To achieve:

- 4000 steps you need about 30 minutes of moderately paced walking

- 7500 steps you need about 45 minutes of moderately paced walking

- 10 000 steps you need about 60 minutes of briskly paced walking

To help you achieve your walking goal, clip a pedometer to your waistband or belt in the morning and start counting. Of course the pedometer only counts steps and not any other activities.

3. Plus planned exercise – it's worth it

Exercise and activity speed up your metabolic rate (increasing the amount of energy you use) which helps you to balance your food intake and control your weight. Exercise and activity also make your muscles more sensitive to insulin and increase the amount of fat you burn.

A healthy low GI diet has the same effect. Low GI foods reduce the amount of insulin you need, which makes fat easier to burn and harder to store. Since body fat is what you want to get rid of when you lose weight, exercise or activity in combination with a low GI diet makes a lot of sense.

Best of all, the effect of exercise doesn't end when you stop moving. People who exercise have higher metabolic rates and their bodies burn more calories per minute even when they are asleep!

If you are ready to improve your fitness, making a commitment to a planned exercise programme including aerobic, resistance and flexibility/stretching exercises will give you the best results. Variety is also important.

Planned exercise doesn't mean having to sweat it out in a gym. The key is to find some activities you enjoy – and do them regularly. Just 30 minutes of moderate exercise each day can improve your health, reducing your risk of heart disease and type 2 diabetes. If you prefer you can break this into two 15-minute sessions or three 10-minute sessions. You'll still see the benefits. Remember, every little bit counts.

What about personal trainers?

Working with a personal trainer can be a great way to improve your health and fitness and work towards your goals. A good trainer will design an exercise programme tailored to your needs and fitness level as well as providing motivation and support. Many personal trainers now provide services for a reasonable rate and you can choose to use a health club or train at home or outdoors. If cost is an issue, you could train with a small group of three or four others with similar fitness levels, or you could just have a few sessions initially. If you can, try to budget for at least 10 sessions. This will help you achieve your goals and increase your confidence with the new exercises.

How to find a good personal trainer

Many trainers are attached to health clubs, but if you don't belong to one or you would prefer to train at home or outdoors, look in your local newspaper or search online for someone in your area. Ask to see their qualifications – they should have at least Level 3 in Instructing Physical Exercise & Exercise. Go to *www.exerciseregister.org* for more information. A good trainer should offer you at least one complimentary session to 'try before you buy'.

What to expect when you see a personal trainer

In your first session, a good personal trainer will ask you about your current lifestyle, your goals and expectations and any health or medical problems. He or she will then work out a programme to help you reach your goals and work closely with you to implement the plan, supervising each of your exercise sessions to make sure you are performing the exercises correctly and pushing you to the next level. He or she will also help to motivate you when the going gets tough.

Health tip:

Did you know that the benefits of exercise don't stop when you stop? People who exercise have higher metabolic rates and their bodies burn more calories per minute – even when they are sound asleep!

Before starting . . .

If you have any concerns about your health, or any illnesses such as diabetes or heart problems or an injury, discuss your activity plan with your GP first.

Here are some ideas to get you started

- aerobics
- aqua-robics
- cycling
- dancing
- exercise balls
- exercise bikes
- exercise classes
- exercise DVDs and videos
- golf
- health clubs and gyms
- paddling, rowing and kayaking
- Pilates
- spin classes
- surfing and bodysurfing
- swimming
- table tennis
- tai chi
- team sports
- tennis, squash and other racket sports
- treadmills
- weight training
- yoga

PART 3

The Top 100
low gi food finder

Everyone can benefit from the low GI approach to eating. It is the way nature intended us to eat – slow-burning, nutritious foods that satisfy our hunger.

To pick the top 100 low GI foods for healthy eating and to give you plenty of choice, we pushed our shopping trolley up and down the supermarket aisles. We have listed the foods in this section A to Z within the appropriate food group to make meal planning and shopping easier.

We are often asked about foods such as lean red meat, chicken, eggs, fish and seafood – foods that don't have a GI because they don't contain carbs. As a result we have also included brief sections on these protein-rich foods because they are an important part of a healthy diet.

The food groups

When planning meals, choose foods from all the groups to make sure you gain the benefits of the 40+ essential nutrients along with the protective anti-oxidants and phytochemicals your body needs each day for long-term health and wellbeing.

We have also included a few 'borderline' low–medium GI foods as they are great additions to your diet.

Which brand?

Low GI eating often means making a move back to staple foods – pulses, whole cereal grains, vegetables and fruit – which naturally have a low GI, so it doesn't matter what brand you buy.

Knowing which brand to buy is important, however, when it comes to choosing carb-rich processed foods such as breads and breakfast cereals whose GI values can range from low to high.

To find the GI of your favourite brands you can:

- Look for a low GI symbol on foods.
- Check the nutritional label – some manufacturers include the GI.
- Visit **www.glycemicindex.com** to search a reliable database of GI values.
- Check the GI tables on page 219.

If you can't find the GI of your favourite breakfast cereal or bread, contact the manufacturer and suggest they have the food tested by an accredited laboratory.

GI values

A low GI value is 55 or less

A medium value is 56–69

A high GI value is 70 or more

Are you eating enough fibre?

Many low GI foods are good sources of dietary fibre, which is a terrific bonus since we need about 18 grams of fibre a day for bowel health and to keep regular. Filling, high fibre foods can also help you maintain a healthy weight by reducing hunger pangs.

Dietary fibre comes from plant foods – it is found in the outer bran layers of grains (corn, oats, wheat and rice and in foods containing these grains), fruit and vegetables and nuts and pulses (dried beans, peas and lentils). There are two types – soluble and insoluble – and there is a difference.

A word on processed food

Try to avoid highly processed foods as much as possible. Think of it this way: you should do the processing, not the food company!

- *Soluble fibres* are the gel, gum and often jelly-like components of apples, oats and pulses (beans, peas and lentils). By slowing down the time it takes for food to pass through the stomach and small intestine, soluble fibre can lower the glycaemic response to food.
- *Insoluble fibres* are dry and bran-like and commonly thought of as roughage. All cereal grains and products made from them that retain the outer coat of the grain are sources of insoluble fibre, e.g. wholemeal bread and

All-Bran®, but not all foods containing insoluble fibre are low GI. Insoluble fibres will only lower the GI of a food when they exist in their original, intact form, for example in whole grains of wheat. Here they act as a physical barrier, delaying access of digestive enzymes and water to the starch within the cereal grain.

FRUIT & VEGETABLES

When it comes to fruit and vegetables think colour, think variety, think protective anti-oxidants, and give these foods a starring role in your meals and snacks.

Fruit and vegetables play a central role in a low GI diet. While we all remember being told to eat our greens, we believe that it's important to eat seven or more serves of fruit and vegetables every day for long-term health and wellbeing. The greater the variety, the better.

Green

- artichokes, Asian greens, asparagus, avocados, bok choi, broccoli, broccolini, Brussel sprouts, cabbage and Chinese cabbage, celery, chard, chicory, courgettes, cress, cucumber, endive, green beans, green peppers, leafy greens, leeks, lettuce, marrow, mesclun, okra, peas (including mangetouts and sugar snap peas), rocket, silverbeet, spinach, spring onions, watercress
- green apples, figs, green grapes, honeydew melons, kiwi fruit, limes, green pears

Red/pink

- red peppers, radishes, red onions, tomatoes, yams
- red apples, blood oranges, cherries, cranberries, red grapes, pink/red grapefruit, guavas, plums, pomegranates, raspberries, rhubarb, strawberries, tamarillo, watermelon

White/cream

- bamboo shoots, cauliflower, celeriac, daikon, fennel, garlic, Jerusalem artichoke, kohlrabi, mushrooms, onions, parsnips, potatoes (white-fleshed), shallots, swedes, taro, turnips, white onions
- bananas, lychees, nectarines, white peaches

Orange/yellow

- butternut squash, carrots, yellow/orange peppers, pumpkin, marrow, sweetcorn, sweet potato, winter squash, yellow beets, yellow tomatoes
- yellow apples, apricots, cantaloupe, custard apple, gooseberries, grapefruit, lemons, mandarins, mangoes, nectarines, oranges, papaya (pawpaw) peaches, persimmons, pineapple, tangerines

Blue/purple

- aubergine, beetroot, purple asparagus, radicchio lettuce, red cabbage
- blackberries, blackcurrants, blueberries, boysenberries, purple figs, purple grapes, plums, raisins

Wash first

Wash all fruit and vegetables before you eat or cook them. If you are going to eat the skins, use a scrubbing brush on vegetables such as potatoes and carrots. For leafy vegetables such as cabbages and lettuce, remove the outer leaves first, then wash leaves individually and dry in a salad spinner.

Why are fruit and vegetables so important?

A high fruit and vegetable intake has been consistently linked with better health. It could be because they are packed with anti-oxidants – nature's personal bodyguards – which protect body cells from damage caused by pollutants and the natural ageing process.

Some key anti-oxidants

Beta-carotene – the plant form of vitamin A, used to maintain healthy skin and eyes. A diet rich in beta-carotene may even reduce damage caused by UV rays. Apricots, peaches, mangoes, carrots, broccoli and sweet potato are particularly rich in beta-carotene.

Vitamin C – nature's water-soluble anti-oxidant found in virtually all fruits and vegetables. Some of the richest sources are cantaloupes, guavas, oranges, peppers and kiwi fruit. Vitamin C is used to make collagen, the protein that gives our skin strength and elasticity.

Anthocyanins – the purple and red pigments in aubergine, blackberries, blueberries and peppers also function as anti-oxidants, minimising the damage to cell membranes that occurs with ageing.

Here's how you can eat seven or more servings of fruit and vegetables a day.

❏ Top muesli or *breakfast* cereal with sliced fruit.
❏ Sip a small juice for a *morning snack.*
❏ Enjoy a vegetable soup or salad for lunch.
❏ Boost your brainpower *mid-afternoon* with a snack such as a handful of grapes or crispbread topped with ricotta and tomato slices.
❏ Brighten your *dinner* plate with a variety of vegetables such as sweet potato, green beans and red and yellow peppers plus a big salad.
❏ Finish your meal with a fruity *dessert* or a fruit platter.

FRUIT

Naturally sweet and filling, fruit is widely available, inexpensive, portable and easy to eat – just like other snack foods, but without the added fat and sugar. So, buy the best you can and enjoy a lifetime of benefits.

People who eat three of four serves of fruit a day, particularly apples and oranges, have the lowest overall GI and the best blood glucose control.

The sugars in fruits and berries have provided energy in the human diet for millions of years. It shouldn't come as too much of a surprise, therefore, to learn that these sugars have low GI values. Fructose, in particular – a sugar that occurs naturally in all fruits and in floral honey – has the lowest GI of all. Fruit is also a good source of soluble and insoluble fibres which can slow digestion and provide a low GI. And as a general rule, the more acidic a fruit is, the lower its GI value.

Temperate climate fruits – apples, pears, citrus (oranges, grapefruit) and stone fruits (peaches, plums, apricots) – all have low GI values.

Tropical fruits – cantaloupe, pineapple, papaya (pawpaw),

banana and watermelon tend to have higher GI values, but their glycaemic load (GL) is low because they are low in carbohydrate. So keep them in the fruit bowl and enjoy them every day if you wish as they are excellent sources of anti-oxidants.

How much?

One serving is equivalent to:

- 1 medium piece of fresh fruit such as an apple, banana, mango, orange, peach or pear (about 115 grams/4 oz)
- 2 small pieces of fresh fruit such as apricots, kiwi fruit or plums (about 60 grams/2¼ each)
- 115 grams (4 oz) of fresh diced or canned fruit pieces including grapes and chopped berries and strawberries
- 4–5 dried apricot halves, apple rings, figs or prunes (about 30 grams/1 oz)
- 1½ tablespoons sultanas (about 30 grams/1 oz)
- 150 ml (5 fl oz) fruit juice, homemade or unsweetened, 100 per cent juice

How much a day?

- Smaller eaters: 2 serves
- Medium eaters: 3 serves
- Bigger eaters: 4 serves

Serving suggestions

1. Fruit is nature's takeaway food. Carry fresh fruit or a small container of fruit pieces or dried fruit to snack on.
2. Top your breakfast cereal with fresh fruit such as berries and sliced bananas or add diced fruit to low fat yoghurt snacks.
3. Whip up smoothies with fresh fruit, juice and low fat yoghurt or make fresh fruit ice-cubes with juice or simply freeze some fruit!

Fruit juice – watch how much you drink

It's all too easy to overdo the calories when drinking juice. For example, if you buy a 'large' orange juice in a café or fast food outlet that offers value-for-money portions, you may find you are consuming the equivalent of ten oranges (3000 kJ/715 Kcal)! Remember, one serving is 150 ml (5 fl oz).

4. Toss fresh fruit slices (apples, citrus segments, strawberries, pears) or whole grapes into crispy green salads. Add a few nuts and serve with a light oil and vinegar or citrus dressing.

5. Prepare a fruit platter (including grapes, strawberries, slices of melon, apple or pear, orange segments, etc.) for dessert or to nibble on while watching television; or keep a bowl of your favourite fruit within reach.

6. It's more likely to tempt you if it's right in front of you, so store fruit or vegetable pieces (such as diced melon or carrot sticks) in a clear container in the refrigerator.

7. Sliced pear, apple, banana or pineapple make great toasted sandwich fillings.

8. Serve fresh fruit salsa with meat, chicken or fish, or use as a salad dressing or dip.

9. Make fruit compotes for desserts or toppings for low fat ice-cream, pancakes and waffles.

10. Try apple or pear slices with some cheese and wholegrain crackers or top grainy toast with thinly sliced peaches, strawberries, apples or pears and a dollop of ricotta or cottage cheese.

> **Thirst-quencher**
>
> Eating fruit regularly is a great way to keep hydrated: some fruits such as watermelon contain up to 90 per cent water. If you're not well hydrated, all your body functions, from joint lubrication and muscle contraction through to digestion and mental performance can be compromised.

APPLES

GI 38

Apples are the ultimate portable snack. It's said that the Roman legions munched them as they marched, the *Mayflower* Pilgrims packed them when they set sail for America, and Captain Phillip stocked up before heading for Botany Bay. Just one fresh apple will give you about one-third of your vitamin C needs for the day and by stimulating saliva it can also help prevent dental decay. Apples are a good source of dietary fibre, particularly pectin, which promotes a healthy balance of bacteria in the intestine. On top of this, apples, particularly the skins, are packed with anti-oxidants.

Simply wash, dry and enjoy as a snack, skin and all

(some people even eat the core), or eat one for a sweet finish to meals. Cooking apples is likely to raise the GI *slightly*.

Serving suggestions

- Add coarsely grated apple to your muesli or favourite low GI breakfast cereal, or to muffin mixes when baking.
- Bake or microwave whole apples for a warm and filling dessert, or core and stuff with dried fruit, a little honey and a sprinkle of cinnamon, then bake.
- Add apple slices to sandwiches and salads or serve apple slices with fruit and cheese platters.
- Slice into segments and use to make stewed apple with cloves, open apple tarts or apple crumbles with a crunchy toasted muesli topping.

APPLE RINGS, DRIED
GI 29

A rich source of fibre, dried apple rings are great for lunch boxes, and a tasty ingredient to chop and add to muesli and other breakfast cereals, fruit and nut mixes, health bars and fruit slices and desserts. Drying concentrates the calories, so count about 10 rings as a serving.

Serving suggestions

- Make a compote by microwaving or simmering dried apple with other fruits and a cinnamon quill in just enough water to cover.
- Soak dried apple in boiling water for about 30 minutes and use in desserts or baking or to make an apple sauce for serving with meat.

APPLE JUICE
GI 40 (unsweetened)

Apple juice is a good source of vitamin C and potassium. The fibre, however, is lost during processing, along with many of the other nutrients in apple skin. When buying juice, look for unsweetened, 100 per cent juice. To make your own, quarter and core two apples and cut into pieces that will fit into the food tube of your juicer, process and enjoy a small glass of juice (150 ml/5 fl oz) as a snack or to finish a meal. Add sticks of celery, carrot or a little fresh ginger for variety.

Serving suggestions

- Sip on a long apple spritzer made with 125 ml (4 fl oz) of juice plus plenty of crushed ice, soda water and fresh mint leaves.
- Make apple juice ice-cubes to cool down on hot days.
- Start the day with muesli moistened with apple juice rather than low fat milk.
- Use apple juice to sweeten breakfast cereal and other foods.

> For maximum health benefits, be choosy about the juice you buy. Look for brands with no added sugar and juices that are pressed whole including the skins, pips and cores.

APRICOTS

GI 57

For fragrance and flavour, fresh apricots are almost irresistible. This sweet 'borderline' low–medium GI fruit is delicious as a snack or to finish a meal. Like all orange–yellow fruits and vegetables, they are rich in beta-carotene and a good source of vitamin C, fibre and potassium.

Cooking apricots draws out their flavour, so they are delicious stewed. If they are not quite ready for eating when you buy them, they should ripen in a day or two at room temperature in your fruit bowl (or in a paper bag away from heat and light). To eat your fill of apricots year round, choose canned or dried apricots. Canned apricots have a medium GI (64). Or, for a delicious topping on grainy toast, use apricot fruit spread (GI 56) in moderation.

Serving suggestions

- Grill apricot halves (stones removed) and serve with custard, ice-cream or yoghurt.

- Halve fresh apricots, remove the stones, stuff with a teaspoon of ricotta and top with chopped nuts.
- Gently poach whole or halved apricots in fruit juice with cloves or a cinnamon quill.

APRICOTS, DRIED
GI 30

Dried apricots can be so more-ish it's often hard to stick to just a handful – five or six halves is the equivalent of a serve. However, if you do overindulge, remind yourself of their health benefits: they are high in fibre, a rich source of beta-carotene and provide reasonable amounts of calcium, iron and potassium.

Dried apricots are a delicious snack food whether you are on the run or desk-bound. They also bring a natural sweetness to many recipes: soaked and pureéd for desserts, added whole to casseroles, or chopped and mixed with couscous or rice as a main meal accompaniment.

Serving suggestions

- Simmer dried apricots in a little water, white wine or fruit juice to soften and plump up and serve on their own or with a dollop of low fat yoghurt or ice-cream.
- Add chopped apricots and other dried fruits to home-made muesli.
- Dice and add dried apricots to the mix when baking fruit slices and cookies.
- Make a Moroccan-flavoured casserole with diced lamb or chicken, onions, dried apricots and spices such as paprika and cumin.

BANANAS
GI 52

Bananas are one of the world's most popular fruits. Eat this versatile fruit raw or cooked; whole, sliced or mashed; or as a snack or part of a dessert, fruit salad or meal. They are also a nutritional goldmine: high in fibre, folate and vitamin C and rich in potassium, which is why sportspeople consume them in great numbers after intense exercise to replace nutrients and help maintain peak performance.

Unlike most other fruit, bananas contain both sugars and starch. The less ripe the banana, the lower its GI – ripening causes the starch to turn to sugars and the GI increases. The starch in raw bananas is resistant to digestion and reaches the large intestine intact, where it is fermented by the resident microflora. The products of fermentation are believed to be important for large intestine health and may reduce the risk of bowel cancer. Cooking bananas increases the GI because it gelatinises the starch so that it becomes easily digested.

> Did you know that if you place bananas in a mixed fruit bowl they'll help other fruit ripen?
>
> To prevent a peeled banana from going brown, brush it with a little lemon juice.

Serving suggestions

- If the bananas in your fruit bowl are looking over-ripe, freeze them in their skins, then peel and add to the blender. They make the most delicious ice-cream alternative for creamy thickshakes and smoothies.
- Enjoy banana custard or ice-cream made with semi-skimmed milk or soya drink.
- Add mashed banana to the mixing bowl for muffins and fruit breads.
- Gently fry banana slices in a little margarine and brown sugar and serve with pancakes or a dollop of low fat yoghurt – or both.
- Bake or steam green bananas (about 30 minutes) and serve as a vegetable accompaniment with barbecued meats.

CRANBERRY JUICE
GI 52 (unsweetened)

Cranberries have earned a reputation for promoting urinary tract health and research is now confirming this. Whole cranberries are an excellent source of iron, vitamin C and fibre and are packed with anti-oxidant power. Cranberry juice is a healthy option but, like all juices, drink it in moderation. Remember, drinking a large glass can mean you are taking on board more energy (calories) than you intended – or need. As an alternative, try a cranberry spritzer with ice and soda.

Berries – enjoy them by the bowlful

Apart from strawberries (GI 40), most berries have so little carbohydrate it's difficult to test their GI. Their low carbohydrate content means their glycaemic load (GL) will be low, so enjoy them by the bowlful. They are a good source of vitamin C and fibre and some berries also supply small amounts of folate and essential minerals such as potassium, iron, calcium, magnesium and phosphorus.

Berries are best eaten as soon as possible after purchase. If you need to keep them for a day or two, here's how to minimise mould. Take them out of the punnet and store in the refrigerator on a couple of layers of paper towel and cover loosely with plastic wrap.

Serving suggestions

❏ Combine your favourite berries with a little caster sugar and a tablespoon or two of balsamic vinegar or a little white wine or orange juice. Let the flavours develop for 30 minutes or so at room temperature then serve.
❏ Top gelato, low fat ice-cream or yoghurt with a spoon or two of berries for a snack or dessert.
❏ Make berry smoothies with semi-skimmed milk, soya milk or yoghurt for breakfast or a meal in a glass when you are on the run.
❏ Purée berries for coulis, salsas, sauces, sorbets and ice-creams.
❏ Serve berries for breakfast with muesli or your favourite low GI cereal and a dollop of low fat vanilla or honey yoghurt.

See also Strawberries (page 127).

Serving suggestions

- Blend a tangy cranberry cooler by combining 250 ml (9 fl oz) of cranberry juice with ½ banana, a tub of low fat yoghurt, 100 g (3½ oz) fresh or frozen raspberries and a handful of crushed ice
- Whip up a creamy cranberry-banana flip for two. Blend 1 small banana with ½ pot vanilla low fat yoghurt, 250 ml (9 fl oz) of cranberry juice and 125 ml (4 fl oz) skimmed milk. Add more yoghurt if you like it when the straw stands up straight!

Citrus fruit – nutritional powerpacks

Citrus fruit – oranges, mandarins, lemons, grapefruit and limes – have among the highest levels of anti-oxidants of all fruit. They are also rich in folate, fibre, vitamin C and vitamin A. We know that oranges and grapefruit have a low GI, while the juice of lemons and limes provides acidity that slows gastric emptying and lowers the overall GI of a meal. Try a fresh squeeze of lemon or lime on vegetables with a twist of black pepper just before serving, or toss salad in a dressing made with oil, lemon juice and salt and pepper to taste.

See Grapefruit (page 118); Oranges (page 122).

CUSTARD APPLES

GI 54

Although you may not find custard apples in your local supermarket every day, the range of exotic and tropical fruits available is on the increase to satisfy consumer demand. In fact, with online shopping options, exotic fruit such as custard apples, which are also grown in Spain, can be delivered to your door. Creamy custard apples, originally from South America, taste like a tropical fruit salad and are virtually a complete low GI food source on their own, providing some protein, carbohydrate and fibre along with many essential vitamins and minerals, including vitamin C, potassium and magnesium.

If you haven't tried this fruit before, choose one that's just soft to touch (like an avocado) without splits or bruises. A few black spots on the skin don't matter. Ripe fruit will yield to gentle pressure and can be kept in the crisper section of the refrigerator for up to two days – but be aware that the skin will blacken. If unripe, store fruit at room temperature until ripe. To eat, simply cut in half or twist open and eat the creamy flesh straight away with a teaspoon discarding the black seeds, or scoop out the flesh and add to salads. The flesh discolours rapidly, so brush it with a little lemon or lime juice if you aren't eating it immediately. Add puréed custard apple to yoghurt or to desserts such as cake, sorbets, parfait and ice-cream for a taste of the tropics. Cooking alters the flavour, so stir segments into savoury dishes or curries just before serving to heat through.

Serving suggestions

- Power your day with an energy breakfast of muesli moistened with fresh orange juice and topped with scoops of custard apple.
- For a meal on the run, sip a custard apple smoothie made with low fat yoghurt and semi-skimmed milk with a little honey to sweeten.
- Sleep soundly after a custard apple egg nog made with low fat milk and honey to taste.

Dried dates update

Dates are one of the oldest cultivated fruits and a staple food throughout the Middle East. Rich in carbohydrate, dried dates are a good source of fibre, minerals such as iron, potassium and magnesium and vitamins B6, niacin and folate. Unlike most fruits they contain almost no vitamin C. It would appear that the GI value of dried dates could vary significantly depending on the variety (and there are approximately 600 varieties).

When dried dates were first tested their GI value was 103. This high value was puzzling and was rechecked a number of times. It may be that the amount of carbohydrate per serve on the packaging label was incorrect. A team in the Faculty of Medicine and Health Sciences at the United Arab Emirates University tested the khalas variety of dates in 2004 and found that the average GI value was 39.

Dried dates are a delicious snack or addition to stuffings, pilafs, muffins and winter warming desserts. Like all dried fruits, a little goes a long way.

GRAPEFRUIT

GI 25

Just half a grapefruit contains about 35 mg of vitamin C, which is almost your recommended daily intake. This is one of the lowest GI fruits and provides some fibre too. Choose fruit that feels 'heavy' for its size – this tends to indicate a thinner skin and plenty of juice. Store in your fruit bowl as they are juicier eaten at room temperature.

Serving suggestions

- Start your day with zest with juicy grapefruit's refreshing tang. Halve a grapefruit, loosen the segments and eat as is, or sweeten with a little sugar or a drizzle of pure floral honey.
- Toss segments in salads with smoked salmon and avocado; prawn and avocado; or Belgian endive, radicchio, beetroot and avocado; or simply add to Asian greens and a citrus dressing.
- Combine with chopped pepper, finely chopped onion and a little chilli for a tangy salsa to accompany barbecued meats.
- Enjoy as part of a winter fruit salad with sweeter ingredients such as oranges and raisins and a drizzle of honey.

GRAPEFRUIT JUICE

GI 48 (commercial)

Cool and refreshing as a snack or after a workout, one small glass of grapefruit juice is rich in vitamin C. The grapefruit juice you buy in the supermarket has a much higher GI than the whole fruit, possibly because manufacturers reduce its acidity to produce a juice with wide consumer appeal. If you squeeze your own grapefruit for juice, however, the GI will be similar to that of whole fruit.

Serving suggestions

- Combine with soda or mineral water for a cool, tangy spritzer.
- Add juice to desserts such as sorbets and mousses.

GRAPES

GI 46 (green)

Grapes are a perfect low GI finger food fruit – grab a small bunch and enjoy as a no-mess, no-fuss snack or with a fruit or cheese platter to finish a meal. They are a good source of vitamin C, provide some fibre and red-skinned grapes contain protective anti-oxidants called antho-cyanins. They have one of the highest sugar contents of all temperate fruits, which is one reason why they make such a good starter for alcoholic drinks – more sugar means more alcohol. The first wine (recorded in Mesopotamia and Egypt around 3000 BC) was probably made by accident by allowing a container of grapes to ferment naturally.

Choose bunches with plump, undamaged fruit (avoid split, sticky or withered grapes) and don't be shy about asking if you can taste-test for flavour.

Serving suggestions

- Top cereal with low fat vanilla yoghurt and a handful of fresh grapes to start the day.
- Put a bowl of grapes on the table after dinner.
- Add red and green grapes to fruit salads and side salads.
- Cool off with frozen fruit skewers – grapes, strawber-ries, banana slices and melon or pineapple chunks make a colourful combination.

HONEY

It could be said that we are all born with 'a sweet tooth'. We don't know why, but it may have something to do with the brain's dependence on glucose as its sole source of fuel. Our hunter–gatherer ancestors relished honey and all sorts of other sources of concentrated sugars such as maple syrup, dried fruits and honey ants and went to great trouble to obtain them. So, if you like to sweeten your food with honey or use it as a spread, you are following a long tradition!

The colour and flavour of honey differs depending on the nectar source (the flowers) visited by the honey bees. We now know from our testing in Australia that the GI of honey can vary too, depending on where the bees have been buzzing. We found that in Australia the lower GI honeys are what are called pure floral honeys (average GI 55) from the blossoms of particular eucalyptus nectar sources rather than the mass market blended honeys from a variety of nectar sources (GI more than 70).

Supermarkets do stock pure floral honeys including Tasmanian Leatherwood Honey (Sainsbury's) and Manuka honey but as yet, we don't know their GI. However, there's no need to go without honey, as a modest serving of 2 teaspoons of even a high GI blended honey, actually has a GL of only 5.

JAM
GI 55 (average)

A dollop (1–2 teaspoons) of jam or fruit spread on grainy bread or toast contains fewer calories than lightly spreading it with butter or margarine. So enjoy a little jam on your bread or toast and give fat the flick.

- Strawberry jam GI 51
- Apricot fruit spread GI 56

KIWI FRUIT
GI 53

The furry kiwi fruit provides plenty of vitamin C – just one will meet your daily requirements. They are also rich in fibre, a good source of both vitamin E and potassium and a moderate source of iron. They are renowned as a meat tenderiser thanks to the enzyme actinidin – simply rub cut or mashed fruit over the meat and leave for about 30–40 minutes before barbecuing or grilling.

The best way to eat them is simply to cut them in half and scoop out the flesh. Alternatively peel and slice or dice and add to fruit and green salads, and fruit and cheese platters, or purée and serve with low fat yoghurt, ice-cream, gelato and sorbets.

Serving suggestions

• Toss kiwi fruit slices with watercress and avocado chunks in a light citrus dressing.
• Bring colour and variety to a cheese platter with slices of kiwi fruit, small bunches of purple–red grapes, dried apricot halves and walnuts.

MANGOES
GI 51

Mangoes are one of the few tropical fruits that squeeze into the low GI range. They are also a rich source of vitamin C (one provides your recommended daily intake) and beta-carotene, and a useful source of fibre and potassium.

This versatile fruit is delicious fresh, sliced and puréed in desserts, or combined with fish, meat, poultry along with flavours such as lime juice, chilli and coriander for main meals. You can even eat them green in Asian-style salads and pickles, although you need to choose the right variety of mango. Ask your greengrocer to recommend a green eating mango or visit an Asian produce store.

Serving suggestions

- Stir-fry strips of duck or chicken breast and make a warm salad tossed with golden mango slices, bean sprouts, chopped onion, chilli, fresh mint leaves and a tangy Thai dressing.
- Combine diced mango with chopped red onion, tomatoes, red pepper and coriander and a dash of lime juice to serve as a salsa with seafood.
- Try chopped fresh mango with a scoop of low fat chocolate ice-cream and an almond wafer for a delicious and easy dessert.

ORANGES
GI 42

One orange is something of a personal protection powerhouse, providing you with your whole day's vitamin C requirement. Oranges are rich in anti-oxidants and are good sources of folate and potassium. Much of their sugar is sucrose, a 'double' sugar made up of glucose and fructose. When digested, only the glucose molecules have an impact on your blood glucose levels. This, plus the high acid content, account for the low GI.

Serving suggestions

- Peel and enjoy the juicy segments with breakfast cereal, as a snack, or as an after-dinner palate cleanser.
- Chop into fruit salads, toss into salads, add to soups or casseroles or to couscous.
- Slice and add to fruit punch.
- Carrot and orange make a great couple – enjoy this perfect partnership in soup, salad or juice.
- Oranges make delicious desserts – jellies, sorbets, souffles, crepes, ice-cream
- Try a citrus salad with orange and grapefruit segments, a can of chickpeas, cherry tomatoes and peppery rocket tossed in an oil and lemon juice dressing.

ORANGE JUICE

GI 50 (unsweetened)

Freshly squeezed juice has most of the health benefits of a whole orange, but lacks the fibre unless you throw in the pulp. Its GI will be similar to that of whole fruit. If you are buying oranges specifically for juicing, choose ones that are firm and heavy for their size.

The juices you buy from the supermarket tend to have a slightly higher GI than the whole fruit because they contain equal amounts of fructose, glucose and sucrose. During processing much of the original sucrose is partially split or 'hydrolysed' to glucose and fructose. When shopping look for unsweetened, 100 per cent juice.

Use orange juice to moisten breakfast cereal as a change from milk, or add to meat dishes, couscous or spinach salads to help increase iron absorption. And remember, it's all too easy to overdo your juice intake – a serve is just 150 ml (5 fl oz).

> **The true pawpaw**
>
> The true pawpaw or papaw (*Asimina triloba*) is a North American native from the same family as custard apples. It has creamy-yellow, sweet flesh with a custard-like texture and looks rather like a fat, brown banana.

Serving suggestions

- Add juice to fruit punches, fruit salad, milk shakes and egg nog.
- Use orange juice's zesty flavour in marinades, sauces and dressings.
- Freeze juice to make summer treats such as ice-lollies and ice pops.

PAPAYA/PAWPAW

GI 56

You can be forgiven for being confused about whether to call this large, oval-shaped tropical fruit papaya or pawpaw, or even whether it's the same fruit, as the names are used interchangeably even by the experts. Native to the Americas, the tropical papaya (*Carica papaya*) is a completely different fruit from Asimina triloba – the true pawpaw (see sidebar). Papayas range in colour from a deep orange to a pale green, and in size from looking rather like a small football to an overgrown pear, depending on the variety. Whichever you buy, however, it will be rich in vitamins A and C, a moderate source of fibre and will have a low–medium GI.

Like many tropical fruits, a ripe papaya is best raw. Simply cut it in half lengthways, scoop out the seeds, peel away the skin, cut the flesh into slices or wedges and enjoy. The green or unripe fruit can be cooked as a vegetable or cut into strips or grated and added to Asian-style salads. The shiny black–grey seeds are usually thrown away, but they are also edible (they have a peppery flavour) – crush them and add to dressings or sprinkle over salads.

Serving suggestions

- Serve papaya slices for breakfast sprinkled with lemon or lime juice for a fresh-tasting start to the day, or dice papaya and add to tropical fruit salads with mangoes, kiwi fruit, passionfruit and berries.
- Purée ripe papaya and use as a sauce or topping or to flavour sorbets and ice creams (but not jellies – fresh papaya will not set in gelatine desserts).
- Serve seafood or chicken with a coriander and papaya salsa.
- Purée ripe papaya and add to marinades (it contains papain, a protein-splitting enzyme which can be used as a meat tenderiser) or just rub a little juice over meat and leave for about 20 minutes before cooking.

PEACHES
GI 42
It's nice to know that something as juicy and delicious as a ripe, fresh peach is so healthy. Peaches are good sources of vitamin C, potassium and fibre.

For eating, look for bruise-free peaches with a fragrant aroma that give a little to touch. For cooking, freestone peaches (ask your greengrocer if unsure) are probably the better choice. The easiest way to peel a peach is to dip it in boiling water, then in cold water. The peel should slide off easily. To prevent discolouration if you are not eating the cut fruit immediately, brush with a little lemon or lime juice.

Canned peaches have many of the nutritional benefits of fresh fruit (with a little less vitamin C) along with a low GI and the convenience of being available year round. Try single serving cans or pots as a snack.

Serving suggestions

- Top grainy toast with ricotta and thinly sliced fresh peaches for an easy breakfast or a tasty snack.
- Halve, stone and poach peaches in champagne, white wine or fruit juice with or without the skin and serve with low fat yoghurt or ice-cream.
- Sip on a fruity whip of puréed peaches or nectarines blended with ice and orange juice.
- Sprinkle fresh peach halves with a little cinnamon and lightly grill.

PEARS
GI 38

Juicy, sweet pears are one of the world's most loved fruits – they've even been immortalised in poetry, paintings and a Christmas carol! They are renowned as a non-allergenic food, thus a favourite when introducing babies to solid foods. An excellent source of fibre and rich in vitamin C and potassium, fresh pears have a low GI because most of their sugar is fructose. Canned pears in 'natural juice' also have a low GI (44) because the fructose remains in high concentration during processing. Single-serve pots and cans are also available. Again, look for those in natural juice.

Although they are often hard when you buy them, pears will ripen at room temperature in a few days. Pack a pear for lunch or to snack on during the day – there's no need to peel as the skin is a good source of fibre.

Serving suggestions

- Dip pear slices in lemon juice and serve with cheese and walnuts.
- Toss in salads – try pear, avocado, rocket or radicchio and walnuts.
- Poach or bake pears in a light citrus syrup or red wine with a touch of cardamom.
- Try topping a bowl of porridge with grilled pear slices and a drizzle of honey or some brown sugar.

PLUMS
GI 39

Plum pudding, plum jam, Chinese plum sauce – this fruit is popular the world over. It's also a good source fibre and provides small quantities of vitamins and minerals. Fresh plums have a low GI and it's likely that canned plums in natural juice will also have a low GI. However they have not been tested yet.

Choose plump, undamaged fruit (no splits, bruises or signs of decay) with a slight whitish bloom and enjoy fresh as a snack or to finish a meal.

Serving suggestions

- Halve, remove stone and add to fruit salads and compotes or serve with cheese or fruit platters.
- Purée for making sauces and delicious sorbets and ice-cream – or plum soup.
- Top stewed plums with a sprinkle of toasted muesli and a dollop of yoghurt for a breakfast with a difference.
- Poach plums in red or white wine with a stick of cinnamon and serve hot or cold.

PRUNES

GI 29

Prunes have a reputation for keeping us regular, but there's more to this tasty dried fruit than that. They are a concentrated source of many nutrients including beta-carotene, B vitamins, potassium and phosphorus. Prunes are also a useful source of iron for vegetarians. Their sugar content, naturally occurring acids and fibre make them a great low GI food for snacks on their own or as part of a fruit and nut mix.

You can buy prunes with stones or pitted – but check for the occasional stone as the processing is not always perfect. Soften or 'plump' by simmering or soaking and enjoy in desserts, or add to lamb, pork, chicken and game dishes for a Moroccan flavour.

Serving suggestions

- Combine prunes with an equal amount of water in a small pan and gently simmer for about 5–10 minutes. Add a slice of lemon or some spices for extra flavour.
- To soften in the microwave, pour fruit juice or water over prunes, cover and cook.
- To soften overnight, place prunes in a heatproof bowl and just cover with boiling water. When cool, cover and store in the refrigerator.

STRAWBERRIES

GI 40

It's no wonder deliciously versatile strawberries are the world's most popular berry fruit. You can eat them fresh, add them to fruit salads and smoothies, use them in a delicious dessert, decorate cakes with them, or make them into jams, fruit spreads and sauces.

Fresh strawberries are rich in vitamin C, potassium, folate, fibre and protective anti-oxidants. Because the average serve has very little impact on blood glucose levels, people with diabetes can eat them freely. So reap the health benefits as you enjoy them by the bowlful, but hold the cream! A word of warning: don't eat too many in a single day. They can have diuretic and laxative effects if you overdo it.

If you aren't eating them immediately, spread the berries out in a single layer on paper towel on a plate and lightly cover with plastic wrap. Remove any damaged or mouldy ones first.

Serving suggestions

- For a perfect parfait, take a tall glass and arrange layers of sliced strawberries, whole blueberries and dollops of low fat vanilla yogurt. Mango slices are delicious with this combination, too.
- Blend strawberries for a bright and refreshing coulis to serve with low fat ice-cream or poached pears. Freeze for fruity ice-cubes.
- Add strawberries to smoothies and shakes with low fat yoghurt or ice-cream.
- Serve whole with fruit and cheese platters or dip in chocolate for a sweet treat with coffee at the end of a meal.
- Quarter fresh strawberries and soak in balsamic vinegar with a little sugar.
- Add to green salads with baby spinach, small cubes of mozzarella and a light balsamic dressing.
- Enjoy a dollop of strawberry jam (GI 51) on grainy fresh bread or toast in moderation.

SULTANAS
GI 56

For a quick and easy low GI snack it's hard to go past sultanas. They are a good source of fibre and also provide some potassium and vitamin E. They are juicier, softer and sweeter than their cousins the currant and raisin, which may account for their popularity in breakfast cereals, muesli and mixes with nuts and apricots. They also make a versatile cooking ingredient – add to all sorts of dishes from casseroles and compotes to couscous, cakes, cookies and crumbles.

Serving suggestions

- A mini-box of sultanas is ideal for school lunch boxes.
- Spread grainy bread with a little peanut butter and make a salad sandwich with grated carrot, cucumber slices, sultanas and shredded lettuce.
- Sweeten breakfast cereal and yoghurt with a spoonful of sultanas.
- Simmer sultanas in apple or orange juice with peeled and grated ginger to make a tasty compote for breakfast or dessert.
- Add sultanas to your favourite bread and butter pudding recipe along with chopped dates.

VEGETABLES

Think of vegetables as 'free' foods – they are full of fibre, essential nutrients and protective anti-oxidants that will fill you up without adding extra calories. And most are so low in carbohydrate that they will have no measurable effect on your blood glucose levels.

Pile your plate high with leafy green and salad vegetables and eat your way to long-term health and vitality.

Leafy green and salad vegetables, for example, have so little carbohydrate that we can't test their GI. Even in generous serving sizes they will have no effect on your blood glucose levels.

Higher carbohydrate vegetables include sweetcorn, potato, sweet potato, taro and yam, so you need to watch the portion sizes with these. Most varieties of potato tested to date have a high GI, so if you are a big potato eater, try to replace some with low GI alternatives such as sweetcorn, sweet potato, yam or pulses. Vegetables such as pumpkin, carrots, peas and beetroot contain some carbohydrate, but a normal serving size contains so little that it won't raise your blood glucose levels significantly.

How much?

One serving is equivalent to:

- About 80 grams (2¾ oz) cooked vegetables (other than potato, sweetcorn and sweet potato)
- 1 dessert bowl of raw salad vegetables
- 250 ml (9 fl oz) vegetable soup (without cream!)
- 250 ml (9 fl oz) pure vegetable juice

How much a day?

Even the smallest eater should aim to eat five or more servings of vegetables every day, including fresh and frozen vegetables, vegetable juices and soups. This is a minimum of 400 grams (14 oz) of cooked vegetables or 4 dessert bowls of salad.

Starchy vegetables – how much a day?

Starchy vegetables such as sweet potato, potato and sweetcorn are higher in carbohydrate so their GI and serve size is more relevant. One serving is equivalent to:

- 1 medium (115 grams/4 oz) potato (a touch smaller than a tennis ball)
- 100 grams (3½ oz) mashed potato
- 115 grams (4 oz) sweet potato
- 100 grams (3½ oz) corn kernels
- ½ cob sweetcorn
- 1 large (about 150 grams/5½ oz) parsnip

In addition to the five or more serves of other fresh or frozen vegetables:

- Smaller eaters: 1 serve
- Medium eaters: 3 serves
- Bigger eaters: 4 serves

Serving suggestions

1. Pile vegetables on your favourite sandwiches. Try sliced peppers, cucumber, onion, tomatoes, broccoli, courgettes, spinach and mushrooms. Or include salad ingredients or chopped up leftover vegetables in a pitta pocket, sandwich or tortilla wrap. Top grainy toast with leftover vegies.
2. Add vegetables to stir-fried meat, chicken, prawns, fish or tofu dishes.
3. Make a meal of stuffed vegetables – peppers, tomato, aubergine and onion all make great 'containers'.
4. Use herbs and spices for flavour and serve two or three portions of different vegetables such as broccoli, carrots and cauliflower or even a ratatouille of mixed vegetables including tomatoes, peppers, aubergine and onions.
5. Throw some vegetables under the grill or on the barbecue with meat. Try courgettes, corn, peppers, mushrooms, aubergine, onion or thick slices of parboiled sweet potato. (Use vegetable oil spray or a little olive oil on a cold grill to prevent sticking.)
6. Make homemade vegetable soups. Try combinations like onion, carrot, celery and tomato in a chicken or vegetable stock. Purée if you prefer a creamy texture.
7. Try a vegetarian main dish at least once a week such as creamy vegetarian lasagne with ricotta, onions, mushrooms, tomatoes, lentils and spinach.
8. Add grated carrot and courgettes to breads and muffins, or grated carrot and onion to rissoles and burgers.

> ### Salad for starters
>
> Enjoy a mixed salad (lettuce, tomato, cucumber, celery, peppers) tossed in an oil and vinegar dressing before moving on to your main course.
> A recent study reported that eating a salad like this for starters helps to fill you up and you will eat less overall.

9. For quick munching, keep celery, peppers, baby carrots, cucumbers, broccoli or cauliflower florets and cherry tomatoes on hand. Dip them in hummous, low fat aubergine or tuna dips or a homemade tomato salsa.
10. Buy a vegetable cookbook packed with recipes you can't wait to try out and buy and try vegetables you haven't cooked before.

Storage and cooking tips

Vegetables are best fresh, so shop two or three times a week if you can and use them within two to three days.

Ethylene gas produced by ageing fruit and vegetables leads to their deterioration. You can minimise the effect of ethylene by storing vegetables in the fridge in long life bags, which are available in the food wrap section of supermarkets, or you can use special cartridges (available in some supermarkets) designed to absorb ethylene. Fruits give off more ethylene than vegetables, but vegetables are more sensitive to its effects so if you have two crispers, keep fruit in one and vegetables in the other.

Wash green leafy vegetables well to remove any soil or grit, then rinse before cooking. They are best steamed or cooked with a minimum of water. Tear salad leaves into small pieces and dry them thoroughly before adding to the salad bowl – the water will dilute the dressing. Salad spinners are great for this purpose, or simply use a clean tea towel.

To make sure you gain the benefit of all those essential nutrients when cooking:

- leave the skins on whenever you can, or peel very finely
- avoid soaking vegetables in water
- use a steamer or microwave for best results
- cook vegetables in big chunks rather than coarsely chopped
- reduce the amount of water you use, cover the pan and

cook quickly and as close to serving time as possible; never add bicarbonate of soda to the cooking water
- cook vegetables until they're softened but still firm to bite

Takeaway tips

When you are ordering takeaway food opt for choices that include vegetables, such as:

- regular hamburger with salad
- pizza piled with vegetable toppings – mushrooms, tomatoes, peppers, spinach, artichoke
- salad with sandwiches, wraps or rolls
- pasta with a tomato-based sauce and plenty of vegetables
- stuffed potato with Mexican-style beans, tomato salsa and cheese
- sweetcorn on the cob
- vegetarian nachos
- salad as a side order or a main course (hold the fries!)
- meat and vegetable fajitas
- corn tortilla with beans and salsa

> ### Salad on the side
>
> A side salad tossed in an oil and vinegar dressing with your meal, especially a high GI meal, will help to keep blood glucose levels under control.

CARROTS

GI 41

'Eating your carrots will help you see in the dark' – sound familiar? Carrots are rich in beta-carotene, a plant form of vitamin A or retinol, which we need to maintain normal vision. A deficiency in vitamin A produces night blindness (an inability to see in dim light). Carrots also provide some vitamin C and fibre, so add them when you're cooking soups, salads, stir-fries, stews, casseroles, cakes and puddings.

Because they make a deliciously crunchy raw snack, it's worthwhile being fussy when shopping and choose firm, bright orange carrots. Avoid the ones with cracks, soft patches or discoloured skin if you can. Grate and add to salads and sandwiches, cut into sticks for dips or snacks, or boil, steam or bake (whole or sliced) and serve with main meals.

Serving suggestions

- Enjoy a freshly grated carrot salad with a bunch of chopped chives and a dressing of oil and lemon juice.
- For a Middle Eastern flavour toss cooked carrot slices in a little oil and lemon juice with roasted cumin seeds crushed in a mortar and pestle.
- Make a creamy, puréed carrot soup with leeks, a potato, and a good quality chicken stock served with a dollop of low fat yoghurt.
- Peel and juice a couple of carrots or add other vegetables or fruit such as celery, apple and orange to start your day with a good healthy glow.

Keep a look out for cassava

Although you may never have seen this starchy tuber in your local supermarket, you may well use one of its best known by-products, tapioca (GI 70), when thickening sauces or making puddings. Cassava (GI 46), also called yuca, manioc and mandioca, is a high carbohydrate staple for millions of people around the world. It looks rather like an elongated potato (about 30 centimetres long) with coarse brown skin and white, fibrous flesh. The roots are usually peeled and boiled, baked or fried. They are also dried and processed into granules, pastes, flours – and even alcohol. The young leaves can be eaten as a vegetable, while the larger, older leaves are sometimes used for wrapping food before cooking.

CORN

See Sweetcorn, page 136.

PEAS, GREEN

GI 48

There's nothing like the aroma of shelling and eating fresh, green peas straight from the pod. Today, most of us buy them in frozen packs – the manufacturer has done the hard work. Green peas are actually a legume, but we have included them here as most of us think of them as a green vegetable. They are rich in fibre and vitamin C and higher in protein than most vegetables. Although a good source of thiamin, niacin, phosphorus and iron when fresh, cooking will reduce the nutrient levels. Frozen peas have about 60 per cent more beta-carotene than fresh peas that have been exposed to light during their trip to market.

If you do buy peas in the pod, you'll need about 350 grams (12 oz) of pods to fill a cup with shelled peas. And tempting as it is to pick up a pack of 'freshly' shelled peas from your greengrocer or supermarket, only do so if you know they really have been freshly shelled and you plan to use them immediately.

Boil, steam or microwave peas for about 4–5 minutes (remember, cooking destroys the nutrients) or add to rice dishes such as risottos, pasta dishes, omelettes, soups and stews (at the last minute), or combine with mashed potato or sweet potato.

Peas with edible pods such as mangetouts and sugar snaps (immature pods) only need the minimum of cooking time, too, and are delicious in stir-fries, or steamed or cooked in the microwave for a side dish.

Serving suggestions

- Whip up an omelette with onion, a little ham or lean bacon and fresh peas.
- If you feel like comfort food, purée or mash cooked peas with chicken stock and a little margarine.

- Add blanched mangetouts or sugar snaps to salads or serve with vegetable platters and dips.

See also Split Peas (page 194).

Have you heard about prickly pear?

The fleshy pads or 'paddles' (nopales) of the prickly pear cactus (nopal) with the spines removed are a traditional ingredient in Mexican cuisine. They are a good source of calcium and vitamin C and contain beta-carotene and iron. They have a small amount of carbohydrate and an amazingly low GI – 7. Sometimes called 'edible cactus', nopales are usually sold in Mexico and the US 'despined' although you'd probably have to trim the eyes with a vegetable peeler to remove any remaining 'prickers'. They can be diced for salads; steamed quickly as an accompaniment (the texture should be crunchy); added to soups, salsas, stews, stir-fries, fillings for scrambled eggs or tortillas; or stirred into Mexican-style recipes with chilli, tomatoes and corn.

SWEETCORN
GI 48 (on the cob)

Sweetcorn is actually the seed of a type of grass that grew in the Americas for thousands of years before Christopher Columbus arrived on the scene. It is rich in vitamin C and a good source of fibre, folate and beta-carotene. It also has higher amounts of protein and vitamin B than most other vegetables because it's actually a cereal grain. Canned and frozen kernels have a similar GI to corn on the cob.

Corn is often used as a base for gluten-free products. However, many products made from corn don't have a low GI at all – cornflakes (GI 77), popcorn (GI 72), cornmeal

(GI 68) and corn pasta (GI 87). Corn chips do (GI 42), but they are also very high in salt and fat.

For the sweetest flavour, buy corn on the cob with the fresh green husk intact, because the natural sugar in the kernels starts converting into starch the moment the husk is removed. To avoid disappointment, stay away from cobs with dry yellow husks and small shrinking kernels.

Boil, steam or microwave briefly, or bake or barbecue and serve piping hot topped with the merest hint of margarine or butter. Toss whole baby corn into stir-fries or cut kernels off the cob (slicing as close to the cob as possible) and add to soups and stews, fritters and frittata, chowders and crepes, salsa and salads. You can substitute canned kernels in recipes calling for fresh, but remember that the flavour won't be quite as sweet.

Serving suggestions

- Spice up barbecue meats with a tangy corn salsa made from diced tomato, red and green peppers, onion, chopped chilli (to taste), fresh coriander and a lime dressing.
- Barbecue cobs by pulling back the husk, removing the silk and then pulling the husk back over the kernels to cover before cooking. When barbecuing, the experts recommend plunging the whole cobs into iced water for an hour before cooking to help the corn cook slowly and evenly.
- Make a sweetcorn frittata with chopped onion, lean bacon, eggs, semi-skimmed milk and parsley and top with a sprinkle of reduced fat tasty cheese.
- Add the finishing touch to a warm salad of roast sweet potato, red onion, red pepper, baby aubergine and baby spinach with small corn cob chunks.

What about potatoes?

Boiled, mashed, baked or fried, everybody loves potatoes. However, we now know that the GI value of potatoes can vary significantly depending on variety and cooking method (GI 56 to 89) – according to University of Toronto researchers reporting in the Journal of the American Dietetic Association in 2005. Their study found that precooking and reheating potatoes or consuming cold cooked potatoes (such as potato salad) reduces the glycaemic response. The highest GI values were found in potatoes that were freshly cooked and in instant mashed potatoes.

In our testing so far in Australia, the only potatoes to make the moderate GI range are tiny, new canned ones (GI 65). The lower GI of these potatoes may be due to differences in the structure of the starch. As potatoes age, the degree of branching of their amylopectin starch increases significantly, becoming more readily gelatinised and digested, thus producing a higher GI. New potatoes are also smaller and there seems to be a correlation between size and GI – the smaller the potato the lower the GI.

Although GI values for potatoes available in UK supermarkets haven't been published yet, there's no need to say 'no' to potatoes altogether just because they may have a high GI. They are fat free (when you don't fry them), nutrient rich and filling. Not every food you eat has to have a low GI. So enjoy them, but in moderation. Try steaming small new potatoes (with their skin for added nutrients), or bake a jacket potato and add a tasty topping based on beans, chickpeas or corn kernels. Add variety to meals and occasionally replace potatoes with sweetcorn, sweet potato or yams, or serve pasta, noodles, basmati rice or pulses.

SWEET POTATO
GI 44

Sweet potatoes aren't a 'potato' at all, they are the roots of a vine from the sprawling morning glory family, and a staple food in many parts of the world. There are several varieties: orange fleshed with red skin (kumara); red-purple skinned with yellow flesh; and white skinned with yellow skin and flesh. All are rich in nutrients including beta-carotene, vitamin C and fibre plus vitamin E, thiamin and folate. A versatile vegetable with a low GI, they make a great substitute for potatoes and, like pumpkin, you can use them in sweet dishes, too. A big advantage over potatoes is that the skin does not develop green patches (which makes them inedible) when exposed to light.

They are as easy to prepare and cook as potatoes – peel or simply scrub the skins and steam, boil, bake or microwave. Try mashing peeled sweet potatoes with a little mustard oil or wrapping small chunks in foil and cooking them on the barbecue. Sliced or cut into chunks, they make a tasty addition to soups, stews, stir-fries and salads (roasted first); cooked and puréed you can add them to scone or cake mixes.

Serving suggestions

- Tuck into a winter-warming shepherd's pie with a sweet potato mash topping.
- Make a spicy stir-fry with onions, ginger, garlic, sweet potato slices, peas and water chestnuts.
- Create casseroles and stews by adding a variety of vegetables including sweet potatoes, tomatoes, onions and carrots to chicken or lean meat.
- Make a creamy soup with sweet potatoes and Granny Smith apples flavoured with cumin and cinnamon and topped with a dollop of low fat plain yoghurt.

Have you heard about taro?

Taro, sometimes called 'elephant ear', is an important food throughout the Pacific Islands. It's a good source of vitamin C and fibre and, like other traditional staples such as sweet potato and yam, it is slowly digested, which is probably why it offered protection against diabetes to at-risk populations such as Pacific Islanders, Maoris and Australian Aborigines. The increased incidence of diabetes in these groups today is linked to increased consumption of modern quickly digested starches.

If you haven't tried taro before, look for firm, hairy tubers with no wrinkling of the skin. Wear rubber gloves when peeling as the juices occasionally cause a skin irritation. Taro flesh is similar to sweet potato in flavour and you can use it the same way – steamed, boiled or cut into wedges and baked.

TOMATOES

As with most vegetables you can tuck into tomatoes without thinking about their GI. They are so low in carbohydrate that they have no measurable effect on your blood glucose levels, but they do provide plenty of fibre, vitamins, minerals and health-giving lycopene, an anti-cancer anti-oxidant.

Products made with tomatoes such as tomato juice and tomato soup are more concentrated and can be a useful source of carbohydrate for light meals and snacks.

CANNED TOMATO SOUP
GI 38

While canned tomato soup is a quick and easy meal with a slice or two of grainy toast, it is also great for quick casseroles and sauces – try it as a bolognese sauce base. Many brands contain large amounts of sodium, so look for salt-reduced ones. A serving is 250 ml (9 fl oz).

COMMERCIAL TOMATO JUICE
GI 38

On the rocks or straight from the can you can feel good about drinking tomato juice (no sugar and minimal sodium added). A thirst-quenching glass provides vitamins A and C, potassium and folic acid. A serving is 150 ml (5 fl oz).

Serving suggestions

- Add beans to your favourite homemade tomato soup recipe and top with finely chopped fresh herbs for a satisfying meal.
- Oven-roast tomatoes and serve with pasta shapes or stir a fresh tomato sauce through spaghetti for a meal in minutes.

Vegetable juices

Watch the sodium content in commercial vegetable juices – look for brands with low- or reduced-sodium labels. Or make your own!

YAM
GI 37

Like sweet potato and taro, yams are high in fibre, nutrient dense and a good source of vitamin C and potassium. They have long been a staple food in Asia, throughout the Pacific Islands and in New Zealand. In Australia the Aborigines ate many species of yam; and when they led their traditional 'bush tucker' lifestyle they were protected from diabetes.

Use yams in your cooking in the same way you would use sweet potatoes, although yams tend to have an 'earthier' flavour. Wash and peel before baking, steaming, boiling or microwaving to serve as an accompaniment or add to salads, soups and stews.

Serving suggestions

- Purée yam cooked with leeks and chicken stock to make a creamy soup and flavour with fresh herbs such as dill or chives.

- Toss cooked bite-sized chunks of yam with mesclun, onion slices, peppers and chives in a light oil and vinegar dressing for a satisfying salad.
- Steam and mash yam chunks with skimmed milk and a teaspoon or two of margarine and season with salt and a few twists of freshly ground black pepper to taste.
- Bake a gratin at 180°C (350°F, Gas mark 4) with over-lapping yam slices moistened with chicken stock, sprinkled with a teaspoon of dried sage topped with grated cheddar cheese and freshly grated nutmeg.

BREADS & CEREALS

High in fibre, rich in nutrients, bulky and filling, wholegrain cereal foods serve us well.

Did you know that the type of bread and cereal you eat affects the overall GI of your diet the most? Why? Well, cereal grains such as rice, wheat, oats, barley and rye and products made from them such as bread, pasta and breakfast cereals are the most concentrated sources of carbohydrate in our diet.

These days, supermarket shelves are packed with products based on quickly digested, high GI flours and grains. Breakfast cereals are a good example. Once, a bowl of slowly digested porridge made with traditional rolled oats gave most of us the energy to keep going from break-fast through to lunchtime. Nowadays we are more likely to fill that breakfast bowl with high GI crunchy flakes that will spike our blood glucose and insulin levels and leave us needing a mid-morning snack to keep going.

A simple swap is all it takes to reduce the GI of your diet. To get started, replace some of those high GI breads and breakfast cereals with low GI carbs that will trickle fuel into your engine. Here's how on the opposite page.

How much?

One serving is equivalent to:

- 1 medium slice bread (sandwich thickness) or ½ English-style muffin
- 30 grams (1 oz) breakfast cereal, rolled oats or muesli
- 100 grams (3½ oz) cooked rice or other small grains such as bulghur or couscous; or cooked pasta or noodles

How much a day?

- Small eaters: 4 servings
- Medium eaters: 6 servings
- Bigger eaters: 8 servings

Switch from this high GI food	To this low GI alternative
Bread – wholemeal or white	Bread and bread rolls containing visible grainy bits, multigrain, 100 per cent wholegrain stoneground, whole wheat, sourdough, sourdough rye, pumpernickel, soya and linseed and fruit breads.
Processed breakfast cereal such as cornflakes and rice bubbles	Rolled oats (not instant), and oat-based cereal such as muesli or a fibre-based cereal such as All-Bran®.
Plain biscuits and crackers; wafers, rice cakes	Biscuits made with dried fruit, wholegrains and oats such as oatcakes, or make your own 'crisp' breads with baked or toasted thin slices of low GI breads.
Cakes and muffins,	Add fruit, oats and wholegrains to the mix. Look for recipes on wholegrain cereal packets. Go halves in a slice of fruit and nut cake or fruit and muesli muffin in a café.
Rice	Choose low GI varieties (basmati or Koshihikari sushi rice) or try buckwheat noodles or barley instead – you can even make a barley risotto.

What's a serving?

A serving is not necessarily the portion you put on your plate. It's a standard reference dietitians use to help give you an idea of the total amount of each of the different types of food you should eat each day. The number of servings you need of particular types of food such as cereal or dairy foods depends on your age and how active you are, and whether you are male or female, pregnant etc.

Serving suggestions

1. Start the day with porridge or muesli, fruit and a dollop of low fat yoghurt.
2. Top grainy toast with creamed sweetcorn, grilled mushrooms or baked beans for something savoury; or ricotta and slices of peaches or apples for a fruity flavour.
3. When buying lunch, choose a grainy or low GI bread or roll for sandwiches.
4. Pack pitta pockets with a bean or chickpea salad, tomato and onion slices and lots of fresh basil or coriander.
5. Serve noodles, pasta, low GI rice, bulghur or quinoa with main meals instead of potato.
6. Add barley, pasta or a low GI rice to soups, stews and casseroles for a filling one-dish wonder.
7. Add bulghur or oats to homemade burger patties or rissoles and serve with a wholemeal bun.
8. Develop a taste for wholegrain bread (try toasting it to begin with), and commit to eating it as your main bread choice.
9. Develop a repertoire of low GI snacks – raisin toast or fruit loaf with a dollop of ricotta; pitta crisps dunked in hummous or salsa.
10. Get hold of a natural wholefoods cookbook, stock your pantry with wholegrain staples and try a new recipe each week.

What about gluten?

People with coeliac disease have a permanent intolerance of gluten, a type of protein in wheat, rye, barley, millet, triticale and oats. Even eating tiny amounts can cause a problem. There are a number of gluten-free products on the market, but with their refined corn or rice starch content many have intermediate or high GI values. If you are on a gluten-free diet and need to reduce the overall GI of your diet, opt for basmati rice or Koshihikari sushi rice, pastas made from soya, noodles made from rice or mung beans and pulses in any form.

Check the tables (page 219) or go to www. glycemicindex.com to find the latest GI values. Or contact manufacturers for information on the GI of their products.

BREAD

Brown or white, wholemeal or multigrain, sourdough or soya and linseed, sliced or in loaves or rolls, bread is truly a staple food – it's inexpensive, low in fat and a useful source of protein, carbohydrate and fibre along with essential vitamins and minerals. In Britain it represents at least 40 per cent of our cereal intake. Most breads sold today have a high GI because they are made from quickly digested refined flours – white or wholemeal. Choose a low GI bread and you are on your way to reducing the overall GI of your diet. Here's how.

Look for really grainy breads, granary, 100 per cent stoneground wholemeal or wholewheat, sourdough, or breads made from chickpea or other pulse-based flours such as soya, or with added soyabeans. Look for these breads in the bread or bakery section of your supermarket, in specialty bakeries or delis, and in health, natural and organic food stores. Check out the ingredient list on the packet. Good choices will list grains such as barley, rye, triticale, oats or oat bran and kibbled wheat; or seeds such as sunflower or linseed; and pulses such as soyabeans. If you want a general rule of thumb: the coarser textured, denser and less processed a bread is, the lower its GI is likely to be.

Don't over-spread yourself

Breads, bread rolls and pocket breads are not fattening in themselves. It's what goes on (or in) them that can pile on the calories. A smear of margarine is all you need – or none at all. For a change, try Nutella®, peanut butter, almond or cashew butter, or avocado. Or you can opt for low fat alternatives like ricotta or cottage cheese or a fresh fruit spread.

Baking your own fruit loaf

As yet we don't have a homemade wholegrain bread recipe with a low GI (although not for the lack of trying). It is very difficult to predict the GI of baked goods that include flour. However, we know that fruit loaves have a lower GI because some of the flour is replaced with dried fruit. This delicious homemade fruit loaf recipe is from *The Low GI Diet Cookbook* (Hodder Mobius). Enjoy it for breakfast, in a bread and butter pudding or toasted as a snack. The loaf is also packed with the fibre needed for a healthy digestive system – 1 slice contains about 4 grams fibre.

To make the fruit loaf put 50 grams (1¾ oz) All-Bran® cereal in a bowl, pour over 300 ml (10½ fl oz) skimmed milk and soak for 30 minutes. Preheat the oven to 180° C (350°F/Gas mark 4).

Sift 225 grams (8 oz) wholemeal self-raising flour and 1 teaspoon baking powder into a bowl and stir in the bran cereal mixture, together with any bran left in the sieve. Stir in 90 grams (3 oz) sultanas, 50 grams (1¾ oz) dried apricots (cut into small dice), 50 grams (1¾ oz) pitted prunes (cut into small dice), 75 grams (2½ oz) dark muscovado or dark brown sugar and 4 tablespoons pure floral honey, and mix well. Spoon the mixture into a non-stick 900 gram (2 lb) loaf tin (or brush the tin with oil to prevent sticking) and level the top. Bake for 1–1¼ hours, or until the loaf is cooked and golden brown on top. Allow the loaf to cool a little in the tin before turning it out onto a wire rack to cool completely.

CHAPATTI

GI 27 (made with besan flour)

Chapatti is an unleavened bread eaten every day by millions of people throughout India and Sri Lanka, and found on the menu in Indian restaurants worldwide. When made with besan flour, chapatti has a low GI. Besan flour is made from ground, dried chickpeas and is also used to make roti and other Indian breads. It's a heavy-textured flour with a distinctive nutty flavour and you can often find it in health food shops, Asian produce stores and the Asian foods section of supermarkets. Nutrient rich thanks to its pulse origins, besan is an excellent source of protein and the minerals potassium, calcium and magnesium.

Chapatti is also made from barley flour and from atta, a wheat flour with a higher GI (63) due to the nature of the starch – so if you are ordering chapattis in a restaurant, ask about the ingredients. If you are making them yourself, use a recipe that specifies besan or gram flour. One chapatti could be equivalent to as much as 3 bread serves, depending on size.

Serving suggestions

- Serve a curry with chapattis instead of basmati rice, or to mop up a delicious dhal.
- Use chapattis to wrap a curry mixture made from lean mince meat browned with your favourite curry paste, a chopped onion and a can of brown lentils or chickpeas. Heat through and stir in a couple of tablespoons of low fat natural yoghurt and freshly chopped mint. Spoon onto one side of the chapatti, roll up and serve while still warm.

FRUIT LOAF

GI range 44–54

There are several types of fruit loaves or breads which include raisins, sultanas, dried apricots or apple, figs and sometimes nuts and seeds. The dried fruit content means they can be a useful source of iron, protein, fibre, thiamin, niacin, riboflavin and magnesium. Generally, the heavier, dense fruity breads will have a lower GI. Enjoy fresh or toasted for breakfast or as a snack.

Serving suggestions

- Snack on toasted fruit loaf with a dollop of ricotta.
- Add flavour to a bread and butter pudding by making it with slices of fruit loaf – great comfort food or for filling hollow legs. Spread 8 slices of fruit loaf with a tablespoon of margarine. Cut into triangles and place in layers in a round casserole dish. Whisk 3 eggs with 500 ml (17 fl oz) of semi-skimmed milk or soya milk and 2 tablespoons of sugar or honey and pour over the bread layers. Stand the casserole dish in a baking pan filled with enough water to come halfway up the sides of the dish. Bake in a moderate oven (180°C/350°F, Gas mark 4) for 40 minutes or until browned on top.

PITTA BREAD

GI 57

Top it, stuff it, wrap it, cut it into wedges and dip it, or split it open and bake it to make 'crisps' – pitta is the ultimate meal-in-a-bread to have around for all occasions. With all the health benefits of ordinary bread, this traditional Middle Eastern flat two-layered bread splits open horizontally, making the perfect pocket for your favourite fillings.

Serving suggestions

- Wrap up with hummous, shredded lettuce, felafel, tabbouleh and a tangy tomato salsa; or avocado, mushrooms, bean salad, shredded lettuce and pepper strips; or tuna, borlotti beans, onion rings, cucumber, feta and a drizzle of oil and vinegar.
- Use pitta bread as an instant pizza base – top with tomato paste, mushrooms, peppers, finely sliced onion, olives and a sprinkle of Parmesan cheese.
- For breakfast, toast and top with fresh light ricotta and a dollop of blackberry all-fruit preserves.
- Serve dips such as hummous and babaghanoush with pitta crisps – simply cut the pitta bread into triangles, open out the 'halves' and spray with a little olive oil, sprinkle over paprika for extra flavour and bake at 180°C (350°F/Gas mark 4) for about 5 minutes, or until crisp.

PUMPERNICKEL

GI 50

This traditional rye bread from Germany can be something of an acquired taste. It's a very good source of fibre and thanks to its high proportion of whole cereal grains, has a low GI value. Also known as rye kernel bread, pumpernickel contains 80–90 per cent whole and cracked rye kernels.

Pumpernickel (no one is quite sure of the origins of the name) has a strong flavour and is dark, dense and compact – not 'airy' like some breads. It is usually sold thinly sliced and vacuum packed for long shelf life. You can crumble it to use in stuffings and for making desserts, but it is most popular as an appetiser.

Serving suggestions

- For an appetiser, top pumpernickel with tangy cheese and apple or pear slivers, spicy sausage and salsa, or smoked salmon, horseradish cream and dill.

Keep them cool

If you plan to make salad sandwiches ahead of time or pack them for your lunch, be sure to include a cold pack. If you're taking your sandwiches on a picnic, park the cooler in the shade. Foods most susceptible to bacteria growth are meats, poultry, eggs and mayonnaise, so be sure they are not left at room temperature for more than an hour.

- For breakfast, toast pumpernickel, spread lightly with margarine and accompany with a hot chocolate drink made with semi-skimmed milk.

SOURDOUGH
GI 54

Crusty, chewy white sourdough's characteristic flavour comes from the slow fermentation process, which produces a build-up of organic acids. It's about the best low GI bread substitute for people who absolutely insist they can only eat white bread. Use for sandwiches and toast (with sweet or savoury spreads and toppings) or serve with main meals, soups and salads.

Serving suggestions
Make bruschetta for a quick and easy light meal or snack. Simply brush slices of crusty sourdough with a little olive oil then lightly grill or bake on both sides and top with:

- fresh tomato and basil salsa with a dash of balsamic vinegar
- char-grilled red and yellow peppers with roasted artichoke hearts
- char-grilled aubergine with semi-dried tomatoes
- mushrooms sautéed with garlic, lemon juice and parsley
- tuna, rocket and capers

SOURDOUGH RYE
GI 54

Sourdough rye is made with rye instead of wheat flour. Slices of chewy, low GI sourdough rye piled with tasty hot or cold fillings make great sandwiches for workdays, picnics or travel. This bread's compact structure keeps the sandwich with all its fillings intact, while the slightly sour flavour combines well with a wide range of meat, poultry, fish and salad fillings.

Serving suggestions

Try these sandwich fillings:

- salad (the works) with rare roast beef and horseradish, or smoked ham and grainy mustard
- smoked turkey with cranberry, avocado and sprouts
- egg salad with fresh chopped chives and crispy cos lettuce
- chicken breast with watercress, apple slices and walnuts
- tuna melt – flaked tuna, finely sliced onion rings and a slice of gruyère cheese
- BLT – lean grilled bacon, lettuce and tomato slices

SOYA AND LINSEED BREAD
GI range 36–57

These moist breads with good keeping qualities are made by adding kibbled soya beans or soya flour and linseeds to bread dough. These phytoestrogen-rich ingredients have been shown to help relieve the symptoms of menopause. They are also rich in omega-3 fatty acids (the good essential oils). Unless you are on a very low fat diet, don't be deterred from enjoying soya and linseed breads as their fat content is unsaturated and they are a good source of fibre.

Serving suggestions

- Club sandwiches; open-faced sandwiches with cold meats and salad and toasted or grilled sandwiches for light meals and lunches.
- For a satisfying salad in a sandwich, skim two slices of soya and linseed bread with a little avocado and fill with a slice of lean ham, tomato, rocket, grated carrot, beetroot, spring onions and sprouts.
- To make a cheesy melt, spread a slice of soya and linseed bread with wholegrain mustard. Add chopped sun-dried tomatoes, grilled eggplant and a slice of mozzarella cheese. Melt the cheese under the grill, top with salad greens and another slice of soya and linseed, slice diagonally and serve.

STONEGROUND 100% WHOLEMEAL OR WHOLEWHEAT BREADS
GI 53

'Stoneground 100% wholewheat bread' means that the flour has been milled from the entire wheat berry – the germ, endosperm and the bran – and the milling process slowly grinds the grain with a burrstone instead of high speed metal rollers to distribute the germ oil more evenly. As a result, virtually none of the nutrient-rich ingredients are lost in the processing, making this bread a rich source of several B vitamins, iron, zinc and dietary fibre. If you can't find stoneground breads in the bakery section of your supermarket, try specialist bakeries or health, natural or organic food stores.

Serving suggestions

- Fill toasted sandwiches with tomato and a slice of cheese or banana, light cream cheese and honey.
- Top toast with a slice of lean ham, spinach, a perfectly poached egg and a drizzle of oil and vinegar.

TORTILLA
Corn tortilla GI 52
Wheat tortilla GI 30

Tortillas are a flat (unleavened) bread traditionally made from corn (maize) flour. A staple of Mexican cuisine, they are quite different from the Spanish tortilla, which is a type of omelette. And when made in the traditional Mexican way, whether from corn or wheat flour, they have a low GI.

Almost any kind of food that does not contain too much liquid – beans, corn or chicken, chilli or salsa – can be placed on or wrapped in the versatile tortilla for a complete meal. Make the most of them with your favourite recipes for burritos, enchiladas, fajitas and quesadillas (but hold the creamy dips) or use as rolls, wraps or scoops. Corn tortillas are also a good alternative to bread if you are gluten intolerant.

Serving suggestion

- To make bean and corn burritos, preheat the oven to 180°C (350°F/Gas mark 4). Combine a 400 gram (14 oz) can of corn kernels, drained, a 400 gram (14 oz) can of red kidney beans, rinsed and drained, 2 large ripe tomatoes, chopped, 2 shallots, finely sliced and 75 g (2½ oz) prepared taco sauce in a bowl. Wrap four 15 cm (6-inch) white corn tortillas in foil and warm in the oven for 5 minutes. To assemble, spread shredded lettuce over a warmed tortilla, and top with the bean mixture and a little grated reduced fat cheese. Fold the bottom of the tortilla over the filling, and roll up to enclose. Serve immediately. Makes 4.

WHOLEGRAIN BREAD
GI range 43–54

Wholegrain breads such as 'multigrain' or 'granary' breads contain lots of 'grainy bits' in the bread (not just on top for decoration). They tend to have a slightly grainy, chewy texture and provide a good source of fibre, vitamins, minerals and phytoestrogens, although this will depend on the flour mix. These are usually made from wholemeal or white flour (or a combination of the two) with kibbled and wholegrains added to the dough.

Choose breads with whole or kibbled grains such as barley, rye, triticale (a wheat and rye hybrid), oats, soya, cracked wheat and seeds such as sunflower seeds or linseeds.

Serving suggestions

- Make your own 'submarines' with wholegrain rolls or muffins
- Top a vegetable gratin with grainy breadcrumbs
- Enjoy a beef or chickpea burger on a grainy bun

BREAKFAST CEREALS

Whether you like waking up to a crisp, crunchy cereal, a warming bowl of porridge or a chewy, nutty muesli, a good breakfast can set you up for the day. Given the solid evidence that people who eat breakfast are calmer, happier and more sociable, the number of people skipping breakfast is an alarming trend. Studies regularly show that eating breakfast improves mood, mental alertness, concentration and memory. Nutritionists also know that having breakfast helps people lose weight, can lower cholesterol levels and helps stabilise blood glucose levels.

ALL-BRAN®
GI 30
With its malty taste, Kellogg's All-Bran® is a good source of B vitamins and excellent source of insoluble fibre. Made from coarsely milled wheat bran, it's among the most fibre-rich of all breakfast cereals on the market. It is also low in sodium and a good source of potassium.

Health tip:

Skipping breakfast is not a good way to cut back your food intake, and it can leave you feeling fatigued, dehydrated and without energy for the day's decisions. Breakfast-skippers tend to make up for the missed food by eating more snacks during the day, and more food overall.

Serving suggestions

- Top a bowl of All-Bran® with banana slices or canned pear slices and serve with low fat milk.
- Sprinkle a few tablespoons over low fat yoghurt as a fibre booster.
- Blend yourself a honey banana smoothie – a cup of low fat milk, a small banana, honey to taste and 15 grams (½ oz) of All-Bran® (or more if you like).
- Add 30 grams (1 oz) of All-Bran® to muffin mixes, banana and other fruit or vegetable breads, biscuits and slices when baking.

BRAN

GI 19 (extruded rice bran)
GI 55 (unprocessed oat bran, average)

You can buy unprocessed oat bran in the cereal section of supermarkets and in health, natural and organic food stores. Its carbohydrate content is lower than that of oats, and it is higher in fibre, particularly soluble fibre. Bran is a soft, bland product useful as an addition to breakfast cereals and as a partial substitution for flour in baked goods to help boost fibre and lower the GI. You can also add a tablespoon or two to meatball and burger mixes, use it in making muesli or add to porridge for extra fibre.

Serving suggestion

Enjoy one of these low GI Cherry Oat Crunchies made with fruit, nuts, oats and bran flakes. Just two delicious biscuits will give you 2 grams of fibre.

Preheat the oven to 180°C (350°F/Gas mark 4). Lightly spray two baking trays with olive oil. Put 55 grams (2 oz) soft brown sugar, 90 grams (3 oz) pure floral honey, 125 grams (4½ oz) reduced fat margarine or butter, 2 eggs, ½ teaspoon of bicarbonate of soda and 2 teaspoons of vanilla essence in a large mixing bowl. Beat using electric beaters on medium speed for 2 minutes. Fold in 150 grams (5½ oz) wholemeal flour, 200 grams (7 oz) rolled oats, 20 fresh cherries (pitted and roughly chopped), 60 grams (2 oz) roughly chopped walnuts and 80 grams (2½ oz) bran flakes cereal, crushed. Mix thoroughly. Drop spoonfuls of the mixture onto the prepared baking trays, spacing them about 5 cm (2 inches) apart. Bake for 15 minutes, or until light brown. Leave for 5 minutes before lifting off the tray and placing on a wire rack to cool. Store in an airtight container. Makes around 42.

MUESLI

GI 49 (natural muesli made with rolled oats, dried fruit, nuts and seeds)

Muesli originated as a Swiss health food, developed by Dr Max Bircher-Brenner who was a passionate advocate of the benefits of a vegetarian, especially raw, diet. It currently rates as one of the few relatively unprocessed breakfast cereals on the market. A good source of thiamin, riboflavin and niacin, its low GI value is the result of the slower digestion of raw oats. Oats also contain fibre that increases the viscosity of the contents of the small intestine, thereby slowing down enzyme attack. This same fibre has also been shown to reduce blood cholesterol levels.

There are essentially three basic types of muesli: toasted, natural (untoasted) and moist (Swiss or Bircher) muesli, but the list of possible ingredients is endless and generally includes:

- cereals: rolled oats, flakes of barley or rice, plus a processed bran cereal if you need to boost the fibre
- nuts: chopped almonds, walnuts, macadamias or hazelnuts
- seeds: sesame seeds, sunflower seeds, linseeds, pumpkin seeds
- dried fruit: sultanas, raisins, chopped dried apricots or figs, pears, bananas, apple rings, cranberries

- spices: cinnamon and other spices are sometimes added for extra flavour

Any muesli will fuel your day, but check the information label when buying toasted muesli as it can contain extra fat and sugar.

Serving suggestion

Try our low GI simple Swiss muesli:

Combine 100 grams (3½ oz) of traditional rolled oats, 125 ml (4 fl oz) of semi-skimmed milk and 2 tablespoons of sultanas in a bowl; cover and refrigerate overnight. Next morning add 100 grams (3½ oz) of low fat vanilla yoghurt, 2 tablespoons of slivered almonds and ½ an apple (grated). Mix well, adjusting the flavour with a little lemon juice if you wish. Serve with your favourite berries – such as strawberries or blueberries. Serves 2.

> Look for breakfast cereals with a 'low GI' label that have been tested by an accredited laboratory such as Sainsbury's Taste the Difference Scottish Jumbo Oats.

PORRIDGE

GI 42 (traditional rolled oats)

The first farmers back in Neolithic times knew that the best way to cook any grain was to make a 'porridge' – all they had to do was crack the grain, add water and cook the mixture in a pot on the edge of the fire. The basic recipe hasn't changed much over the years. The classic porridge we associate with Scotland was made from stone-ground oats simmered in milk or water until cooked, and served with salt or sugar and milk.

For a high-energy breakfast it's hard to go past porridge made with traditional oats – a good source of soluble fibre, B vitamins, vitamin E, iron and zinc. The GI value for porridge has been tested on a number of occasions and the published values range from 42 (for rolled oats made with water) to 82 (for instant oats).

Traditional rolled oats are hulled, steamed and flattened, which makes them a 100 per cent wholegrain cereal. The additional flaking to produce quick cooking or 'instant' oats not only speeds up cooking time, it increases the rate of digestion and the GI. This is why traditional rolled oats are preferred over instant in the low GI diet.

Porridge gourmets advocate steel-cut oats – the wholegrains are simply chopped into chunks. These oats are hard to find but worth the hunt if you like a chewier porridge – and it has a GI value of 51.

Follow the instructions on the packet (or use your favourite recipe) to make porridge. A fairly standard rule is one part rolled oats to four parts water. Cooking oats in milk (preferably semi-skimmed or skimmed) not only produces a creamy dish but supplies you with calcium and reduces the overall GI.

Serving suggestions

Don't skimp on the finishing touches for perfect porridge. Choose toppings such as:

- fresh fruit slices in season
- mixed berries
- unsweetened canned plums
- a teaspoon or two of maple syrup
- a tablespoon or two of dried fruit such as sultanas or chopped apricots

NOODLES

Noodles have long been a staple food in China, Japan, Korea and most of South-east Asia. Today, their meals-in-minutes value has made them popular worldwide – they are a great stand-by for quick meals. They are also a good source of carbohydrate, provide some protein, B vitamins and minerals and will help to keep blood glucose levels on an even keel.

Noodles are made from flour, water and sometimes egg which is mixed into a dough, rolled out to the appropriate thickness and cut into long ribbons, strips and strings – long noodles symbolise long life. Their dense texture and shape whether they are made from wheat flour, buckwheat, mung beans, soyabeans, rice or sweet potatoes contribute to their low to intermediate GI values (33 to 62). Choose lower GI noodles for everyday use.

You can buy noodles fresh, dried or boiled (wet). Fresh and boiled noodles will be in the refrigerator cabinets in your supermarket or Asian grocery store. Use them as soon as possible after purchase or store in the refrigerator for a day or two.

Dried noodles are handy to have in the larder for quick and easy meals in minutes. They will keep for several months, provided you haven't opened the packet.

Egg noodles are made from wheat flour and eggs. They are readily available dried, and you can find fresh egg noodles in the refrigerator section of the supermarket or Asian grocery store. Hokkien noodles are 'wet' egg noodles and will be in the refrigerator section too. Instant noodles are usually precooked and dehydrated egg noodles. Check the label as they are sometimes fried.

Served with fish, chicken, tofu or lean meat and plenty of vegetables, a soup, salad or stir-fry based on noodles gives you a healthy balance of carbs, fats and proteins plus some fibre and essential vitamins and minerals. Enjoy them hot or cold in soups, salads and stir-fries. If they are served crisp, it means that they have been deep-fried.

To cook, follow the instructions on the packet as times vary depending on types and thickness. Some noodles only need swirling under running warm water to separate, or soaking in hot (but not boiling) water to soften before you serve them or add to stir-fries. Others need to be boiled. Like pasta, they are usually best just tender, almost *al dente*, so keep an eye on the clock.

As it's all too easy to slurp, gulp, twirl and overeat noodles, keep those portion sizes moderate. While they are a low GI choice themselves, eating a huge amount will have a marked effect on your blood glucose. Instead of piling your plate with noodles, serve plenty of vegetables – a cup of noodles combined with lots of mixed vegetables can turn into three cups of a noodle-based meal and fit into any adult's daily diet.

Remember when planning meals that the sauces you serve with noodles and how you cook them can provide a lot more calories than the noodles themselves.

BUCKWHEAT NOODLES
GI 46 (soba noodles)

Japan's soba noodles are rather like spaghetti in both colour and texture. They are usually made from a combination of buckwheat and wheat flour and are a better source of protein and fibre than rice noodles. You can buy them fresh or dried, but fresh is better if available. Serve soba hot or cold. One of the classic soba recipes is zaru soba, in which boiled soba noodles are eaten cold with a soy dipping sauce.

Serving suggestions

- For a satisfying pork and noodle soup, season a pork fillet with freshly ground Szechuan pepper then sear on all sides in a little vegetable oil, to get a crust. Cook about 200 grams (7 oz) of buckwheat noodles following the instructions on the packet then drain and add to 2 cups of simmering chicken stock. Stir in a seeded and sliced dried red chilli, 100 grams (3½ oz) of thinly sliced shiitake mushrooms and 2 teaspoons of mushroom soy sauce. Add the thinly sliced pork, a handful of coriander leaves, heat through and serve.
- Make a buckwheat noodle salad by tossing 400 grams (14 oz) of cooked noodles in a dressing made with

about 1 tablespoon of light soy sauce, 2 tablespoons of white wine vinegar, 1 teaspoon of sesame oil, 2 teaspoons of rice wine, ½ teaspoon of finely chopped ginger, 1 clove of crushed garlic and a pinch of chilli (or to taste). Top with finely chopped spring onions and serve. If you like, add thinly sliced pieces of fresh bean curd, too.

CELLOPHANE NOODLES
GI 33

Cellophane noodles, also known as Lungkow bean thread noodles or green bean vermicelli, are fine, translucent threads made from mung bean flour, which is why they have the lowest GI value of noodles tested to date. When soaked they become shiny and slippery and are sometimes called slippery noodles or glass noodles. They are often used in soups, salads and stir-fries. They can also be deep fried. To soften simply soak them in hot (not boiling) water for a couple of minutes before adding them to the dish.

Serving suggestions

- Make a spiced seafood salad using seafood mix from the fish shop (including calamari, crab meat and prawns) with cellophane noodles, chopped Asian greens, mangetouts and a chilli-lime dressing.
- Use leftover chicken to whip up a salad with noodles, blanched mangetouts, blanched green beans, rocket and a light sesame and hoi sin dressing.

INSTANT NOODLES
GI 46

Asian-style dried noodles are very popular as a quick meal or snack. They are a high-carbohydrate convenience food but they also contain a substantial amount of fat – over 35 per cent of their calories in fact. The flavour sachets supplied tend to be based on salt and flavour enhancers, including monosodium glutamate. Keep them for occasional use and add fresh or frozen chopped vegetables when preparing. These noodles can also be added to soups and stir-fries.

Serving suggestions

- For a meal in minutes, make a quick Thai noodle curry. Stir-fry sliced onion, red pepper, baby corn, broccoli florets and mangetouts in a large pan or wok. Add a tablespoon of Thai red curry paste. Prepare instant Asian noodles according to the instructions on the packet. Add to the vegetables with enough stock to make a sauce. Stir in a tablespoon of light coconut milk, heat through and serve.
- Make up a single-serve packet of quick-cook noodles with half the flavour sachet. Add a couple of tablespoons each of frozen peas and corn kernels and then microwave to heat through.

RICE NOODLES
GI 40 (fresh)

Made from ground or pounded rice flour, rice noodles are available fresh and dried. Run hot water through fresh rice noodles to loosen them then drain and combine with other ingredients. Dried rice noodles are rather brittle and need to be soaked for 10 to 15 minutes before adding to soups, salads and stir-fries.

Serving suggestions

- Enjoy rice noodles in broth served with a little lean meat, chicken or tofu and vegetables including chopped Asian greens, bean sprouts, mint leaves and some finely sliced chilli.
- Make up some fresh rice paper rolls: mix together

softened chopped rice vermicelli with grated carrot, fresh bean sprouts, chopped roasted peanuts (unsalted), chopped fresh mint and coriander or parsley and a dressing of sesame oil and lime juice with minced garlic, chilli and a pinch of sugar. Roll up spoonfuls of the mixture in softened rice paper rounds and serve alongside sweet chilli sauce for dipping.

WHEAT FLOUR NOODLES

GI 62 (udon noodles)

Japanese udon noodles are white and usually firmer and thicker than soba noodles. They are available dried, ready boiled and fresh. Cook them according to the instructions on the packet as times will vary depending on the type. Enjoy them hot in soup or cold with dipping sauces and salads.

Serving suggestions

- Combine cooked udon noodles with seared tuna and cucumber slices and toss in a tangy dressing made with soy sauce, lime juice, sesame oil and a dash of wasabi.
- Serve cooked udon noodles cold with a dipping sauce made from soy sauce, mirin and Japanese dashi soup stock and other accompaniments such as sesame seeds, grated fresh ginger, dried seaweed, chopped green onion and wasabi.

PASTA

It's said that pasta (Italian for 'dough') comes in more shapes and sizes than there are days of the year. Whatever the shape, it's perfect for quick meals and scores well nutritionally as a good source of protein, B vitamins and fibre. Pasta in any shape or form has a relatively low GI (30 to 60) –

Al dente

Cooked *al dente*, pasta does not cause sugar spikes when you eat *moderate* portions. *Al dente* ('firm to the bite') is the best way to eat pasta – it's not meant to be soft. It should be slightly firm and offer some resistance when you are chewing it. Its GI is lower, too – overcooking boosts the GI. Although most manufacturers specify a cooking time on the packet, don't take their word for it. Start testing about 2–3 minutes before the indicated cooking time is up.

great news for pasta lovers, but portion size is important. Keep it moderate.

Initially we thought that pasta's low GI was due to its main ingredient, semolina (durum or hard wheat flour). Scientists have now shown, however, that even pasta made with plain wheat flour has a low GI and the reason for the slow digestion is the physical entrapment of ungelatinised starch granules in a spongelike network of protein (gluten) molecules in the pasta dough. Pasta and noodles are unique in this regard. Adding egg to the dough lowers the GI further by increasing the protein content.

As a general rule, commercial dried pasta is made from durum wheat semolina and no eggs; commercial fresh pasta is made with durum wheat semolina and eggs. Homemade pasta tends to be made with plain wheat flour and eggs. There is also some evidence that thicker types of pasta tend to have a lower GI than thinner types perhaps due to their dense consistency and because they cook more slowly (and are less likely to be overcooked).

A number of pasta shapes and types have been tested. Note that canned spaghetti in tomato sauce and packet mix macaroni cheese are not low GI – they have medium to high GI values.

Watch that glucose load. While pasta is a low GI choice, eating too much will have a marked effect on your blood glucose. That's because if you eat too large a portion of even a low GI food the glucose load becomes too large. So, instead of piling your plate with pasta, fill it with vegetables – a cup of cooked pasta combined with plenty of mixed vegetables can turn into three cups of a pasta-based meal and fit easily into any adult's daily diet.

A moderate portion of pasta served with vegetables or tomato sauce or accompaniments such as olive oil, fish and lean meat, plenty of vegetables and small amounts of cheese provides a healthy balance of carbs, fats and proteins.

Pasta salads are ideal for people with busy lives. You can make them in minutes, or prepare beforehand and keep in the fridge until serving time.

Gluten free

These versatile products can be served with sauces, vegetables and used as the basis for salads. Gluten-free pastas based on rice and corn (maize) have moderate to high GI values.

CAPPELLINI

GI 45

This is the thinnest form of pasta (cappellini literally means 'fine hairs') and is made from semolina. Angel-hair pasta is similar in shape, but its dough is made with eggs. Because cappellini is so thin, it is all too easy to overcook it. For a perfect *al dente* product, the optimal cooking time is around 4 minutes. Cappellini comes fresh or dried and is best served with light, smooth or spicy sauces such as tomato, marinara or pesto.

Serving suggestion

A basic marinara sauce is essentially tomatoes and garlic to which seafood (most often these days) is added. To make a basic marinara, cook 2 cloves of crushed garlic and a finely sliced onion in a little olive oil until soft and golden. Add chopped fresh herbs such as parsley and basil (about 4 tablespoons), 2 x 400 gram (14 oz) cans of Italian tomatoes, a splash of white wine, a pinch of sugar and salt and freshly ground black pepper to taste. Simmer uncovered until the sauce is thick, rich and red – about half an hour. Add 250 grams (9 oz) of green prawns (shelled and deveined) towards the end of the cooking time. Cook until the prawns lose their translucency – just a few minutes depending on the size. Makes about 3 cups of sauce.

FETTUCCINE
GI 40

This is the familiar flat, long, ribbon-shaped pasta usually about ½ cm (¼ in) wide. Fettuccine is the term that Romans use for 'noodles'. It's made from semolina and other ingredients such as spinach, squid ink, tomato paste and even cocoa. Available fresh and dried, it's best with tomato- or cheese-based sauces.

Serving suggestions

- Toss cooked fettuccine in a tablespoon of pesto with diced tomatoes and top with a little grated Parmesan cheese. Try using a sundried tomato pesto as an alternative and topping with some pitted black olives.
- Fettuccine is delicious with seafood. While the pasta is cooking, combine a little finely chopped garlic, chopped red chillies and flat leaf parsley in a bowl (adjust the quantity to suit your tastebuds). Pan-fry about four scallops per person in a little olive oil for 2–3 minutes, then add the garlic mixture and heat through. Stir in the drained pasta and serve topped with more freshly chopped parsley.

LINGUINE
GI 46 (thick)
GI 52 (thin)

With its flat shape, linguine is great with many kinds of pasta sauces – pesto and clam or seafood sauces are ideal. It's available fresh and dried and in a variety of flavours including spinach and wholemeal.

Serving suggestions

- Toss *al dente* linguine with peppery baby rocket (stems removed), halved or quartered baby tomatoes, canned tuna and a little oil and lemon juice. Season with salt and freshly ground black pepper and serve warm topped with a little freshly grated Parmesan.

- Red pesto is a piquant coating sauce for all kinds of pasta shapes and ribbons. Combine the following ingredients in a food processor and blend: 15 grams (½ oz) of drained anchovy fillets, a clove of crushed garlic, a tablespoon of toasted pine nuts, a tablespoon of dried breadcrumbs (from grainy bread), a 180 gram (6½ oz) can of red pimiento (drained) or a small jar of roasted peppers, 1 large peeled and seeded tomato, 2 teaspoons of capers, 1 teaspoon of dried oregano and 1 tablespoon of chopped fresh parsley. Add 2 tablespoons of red wine and blend. Slowly add about ½ cup of olive oil and blend in bursts until the sauce has the consistency of pesto. Makes about 1 cup.

MACARONI
GI 47

These short, hollow pasta tubes of 'macaroni cheese' fame combine well with tomato- or other vegetable-based sauces. They are often used in baked dishes, soups and salads.

Serving suggestions

To make macaroni cheese, preheat the oven to 180°C (350°F, Gas mark 4) then cook 400 grams of macaroni following the instructions on the packet. Combine a 250 gram (14 oz) tub of ricotta with 300 ml (10½ fl oz) of semi-skimmed milk, 2 beaten eggs, 2 teaspoons of smooth Dijon mustard, 1 teaspoon of Tabasco sauce (or to taste) and freshly ground black pepper in a food processor and blend. Combine the cooked macaroni with 200 grams (7 oz) of shredded low fat tasty cheddar cheese and 2 handfuls of baby spinach leaves in a bowl. Stir in the ricotta mixture then spoon into a baking dish. Top with grated Parmesan cheese, grainy breadcrumbs and a little paprika and bake for 20–25 minutes. Serve with a crispy green salad. Serves 4.

PASTINA
GI 38 (star shaped)

Small pasta or 'pastina' comes in many shapes: stars, orzo, acini di pepe, and many more. But just like the larger pasta shapes, pastina is made from durum wheat semolina. It is used in vegetable, chicken and beef soups to provide some bulk and added calories to the soup. Children particularly love the shapes of these smaller pastas.

Serving suggestion
Cook 100 grams (3½ oz) of pastina according to the packet instructions and drain. Heat 6 cups of chicken stock and add the cooked pasta plus 2 cups of cooked shredded chicken fillet. Season with salt and freshly ground black pepper and serve with a little grated Parmesan cheese and chopped flat leaf parsley.

RAVIOLI
GI 39 (meat-filled)

Ravioli are small, square pasta 'pillows' with fillings such as meat, cheese and spinach, mushroom, pumpkin and tofu. Buy them fresh, frozen or vacuum packed and serve with a sauce that brings out the flavour of the fillings.

Serving suggestions

- A homemade tomato and basil sauce with a sprinkle of Parmesan cheese is a classic ravioli dish. What makes it even better is that by adding a large salad and fruit dessert you will have created a low GI meal in less than 20 minutes!
- Top a homemade tomato and basil soup with floating ravioli and grated Parmesan cheese.

SPAGHETTI

GI 44 (plain)

GI 42 (wholemeal)

Probably the most popular pasta of all, spaghetti's round, long strands are available fresh and dried and in a variety of flavours such as spinach and wholemeal. With its sturdy texture, spaghetti's versatility is endless. It blends beautifully with cooked and raw vegetables; any mixture of herbs and spices; meats, poultry, fish and shellfish; sauces containing olive oil, margarine, butter or light cream; and even nuts such as walnuts, pine nuts and sunflower seeds – all of which fit in a healthy, balanced diet.

All the low GI virtues of regular spaghetti apply to wholemeal spaghetti and they can be used interchangeably in any recipe with the same sauces and accompaniments. Just keep in mind that you'll be taking in more than double the amount of dietary fibre when you opt for wholemeal spaghetti.

Serving suggestions

• Serve spaghetti with a low fat meat sauce made from lean cuts of beef, pork or veal plus chopped tomatoes, carrots, onions, celery and fresh herbs.

• Toss al dente spaghetti with smoked salmon, capers and a little olive oil and finish with a twist of two of lemon juice.

• Make a spaghetti and tomato salad – enjoy as a light meal and use leftovers for lunch the next day. Dice 3 medium tomatoes and combine in a bowl with 1 tablespoon of olive oil, 1 tablespoon of capers, 1 crushed garlic clove, the juice of a lemon, a sprinkle of chilli powder (or to taste), a few pitted black olives, freshly ground black pepper to taste and a handful of torn basil leaves. Combine with a cup of cooked spaghetti and serve cold or warm. Serves 2.

SPIRALI
GI 43

There are so many dried pasta shapes – from spirals (spirali), shells (conchiglie), bows (farfalle, literally butterflies), quill-shaped tubes (penne and penne rigate), small wheels (rotelle), twists (gemelli, literally twins) to round tubes such as cannelloni which are stuffed then baked. Everyone has their favourites. The great news for pasta lovers is that they all have a relatively low GI. Whether you serve them with tomato- or vegetable-based sauces, simply fold through your favourite vegetables or use them in salads, they are ideal for creating healthy, balanced meals in minutes.

Serving suggestions

- Serve your favourite shapes with lightly steamed cauliflower or broccoli florets and diced lean crispy bacon (pancetta is even better) cooked with a sliced red chilli. Top with chopped parsley and a little grated Parmesan.
- Enjoy a quick pasta and red bean salad. Combine 200 grams (7 oz) of cooked pasta shapes with 200 grams (7 oz) of canned red kidney beans (drained), 3 finely chopped spring onions and a tablespoon of chopped fresh parsley. Toss with an oil and vinegar dressing made from 1 tablespoon of olive oil, 1 tablespoon of white wine vinegar, 1 teaspoon of Dijon mustard, a crushed clove of garlic and freshly ground black pepper. Serves 4.

TORTELLINI
GI 50 (cheese)

Tortellini are a small, crescent-shaped, filled pasta available in a range of fillings – including spinach and ricotta, chicken, veal, ham, mushrooms and cheese in a variety of combinations. The overall nutrient content will vary depending on the fillings. You can usually buy it fresh, frozen or vacuum packed and all you have to do is cook and serve.

Serving suggestions

- Toss cooked tortellini with fresh chopped herbs such as parsley and basil, a minced garlic clove and a little olive oil.
- Try this time-saving tortellini meal. Cook spinach and cheese tortellini according to the packet instructions until al dente and serve with bought or homemade tomato sauce topped with a little grated Parmesan cheese. Serve with a big garden salad for a complete meal in minutes.

VERMICELLI
GI 35
Rather like cappellini, vermicelli is a thin type of spaghetti that's available fresh and dried. Because it is so fine it cooks quickly, so watch the times. Serve with light sauces or add to soups and stir-fries.

Serving suggestions
Toss *al dente* vermicelli with:

- lightly steamed strips of courgette, finely chopped parsley, a few walnut halves, a twist of black pepper and a little grated Parmesan cheese
- a bought or homemade tomato sauce with yellow and red marinated pepper slices, anchovies, flaked canned tuna, olives, capers and basil

Pasta makes a quick and easy meal with many prepared pasta sauces on the market (although it's easy to make your own). Stick to tomato-based sauces or toss with vegetables rather than the creamy ones laden with fat. And use a modest sprinkle of cheese on top.

RICE

Carb-rich rice is one of the world's oldest and most culti-vated grains – there are some 2000 varieties worldwide – and the staple food for over half the world's population. A soup, salad or stir-fry based around rice with a little fish, chicken, tofu or lean meat and plenty of vegetables will give you a healthy balance of carbs, fat and protein plus some fibre and essential vitamins and minerals.

Rice can have a very high GI value, or a low one, depending on the variety and its amylose content. Amylose is a kind of starch that resists gelatinisation. Although rice is a wholegrain food, when you cook it, the millions of microscopic cracks in the grains let water penetrate right to the middle of the grain, allowing the starch granules to swell and become fully 'gelatinised', thus very easy to digest.

So, if you are a big rice eater, opt for the low GI vari-eties with a higher amylose content such as basmati or Koshihikari (Japanese sushi rice). These high-amylose rices that stay firm and separate when cooked combine well with Indian, Thai and Vietnamese cuisines.

Brown rice is an extremely nutritious form of rice and contains several B vitamins, minerals, dietary fire and protein. Chewier than regular white rice, it tends to take about twice as long to cook. The varieties available in Britain that have been tested to date have a high GI, so enjoy it occasionally, especially combined with low GI foods. Arborio risotto rice releases its starch during cooking and has a medium GI. Wild rice (GI 57) is not actually rice at all, but a type of grass seed.

As with pasta and noodles, it's all too easy to overeat rice, so keep portions moderate. Even when you choose a low GI rice, eating too much can have a marked effect on your blood glucose. A cup of cooked rice combined with plenty of mixed vegetables can turn into three cups of a rice-based meal that suits any adult's daily diet.

Why 'gelatinisation' means high GI

The starch in raw carb-rich foods such as rice grains is stored in hard, compact granules that make the food difficult to digest unless you cook it. This is why eating raw potatoes can give you a stomach ache. During cooking, water and heat expand starch granules to different degrees; some actually burst and free the molecules. This happens when you make gravy by heating flour and water until the starch granules burst and the gravy thickens. If most of the starch granules have swollen during cooking, we say that the starch is fully gelatinised. It is now also easy to digest, which is why the food will have a high GI.

BASMATI RICE
GI 58

Basmati is a long grain aromatic rice grown in the foothills of the Himalayas and is especially popular in India. When cooked the grains are dry and fluffy, so they make the perfect bed for curries and sauces. You can buy brown or white basmati rice – brown basmati has more fibre and a stronger flavour, but it takes twice as long to cook. It also has a higher GI.

Serving suggestions

- Toss rice in an oil and vinegar dressing with sultanas, chopped red and green peppers, sweetcorn kernels and finely sliced red onion and celery to make a simple salad.
- Rice on the run is great for lunch the next day, too. Pour a lightly beaten egg into an oiled frypan and cook over a medium heat until bubbly. Flip over to cook on the other side, turn onto a board and chop into slices. Sauté a finely diced courgette and a red pepper, a stick of thinly sliced celery and a grated carrot in a little oil

> Freshly cooked rice has a higher GI than cold, reheated rice. This is one of the reasons for sushi's low GI.

in the pan. Add minced garlic, ginger and chopped shallots, stir till aromatic, then add 100 grams (3½ oz) of cooked basmati rice and stir until heated through. Sprinkle with soy sauce to serve.

SUSHI
GI 48–55

Ideal for snacks and light meals, these bite-sized parcels are usually made with combinations of raw or smoked fish, chicken, tofu and pickled, raw and cooked vegetables and wrapped in dried seaweed and rice seasoned with vinegar, salt and sugar. Even though the rice used to make sushi is short grain and somewhat sticky, sushi still has a low GI, possibly because of the vinegar (acidity puts the brakes on stomach emptying) and the viscous fibre in the dried seaweed. In addition, sushi made with salmon and tuna boosts your intake of healthy omega-3 fats. Sushi served with miso is a delicious light and low GI lunch.

In Japan, sushi is made with Koshihikari rice (GI 48), a short grain rice also called sushi rice with an appetising aroma, sweet flavour, a lightly sticky, soft texture when cooked and a low GI. Use it whenever a softer textured rice is required such as in desserts. You can also use it as a low GI substitute for arborio rice when making a risotto.

Serving suggestions

- It is perfect for sushi, rice balls and other Japanese and Korean dishes, but Koshihikari also goes well with all Asian food.
- Koshihikari makes delicious rice puddings or creamed rice. Boil ½ cup of rice with 1 cup of water for 5 minutes until the water is absorbed. Add 2 cups of low fat milk and cook over a low heat for 20–25 minutes until the rice is tender. Stir in sugar, honey or other sweetener to taste.

WHOLE CEREAL GRAINS

Wholegrain simply means grains that are eaten in nature's packaging – or close to it – traditional rolled oats, cracked wheat and pearl barley, for example. The slow digestion and absorption of these foods will trickle fuel into your engine at a more usable rate and therefore keep you satisfied for longer.

There are countless reasons to include more whole cereal grains in your diet, but it's hard to go past the fact that because you are eating the whole grain, you get all the benefits of its vitamins, minerals, protein, dietary fibre and protective anti-oxidants. Studies around the world show that eating plenty of wholegrain cereals reduces the risk of certain types of cancer, heart disease and type 2 diabetes.

A higher fibre intake, especially from whole cereal grains, is linked to a lower risk of cancer of the large bowel, breast, stomach and mouth. Eating these higher fibre foods can help you lose weight because they fill you up sooner and leave you feeling full for longer. They improve insulin sensitivity, too, and lower insulin levels. When this happens, your body makes more use of fat as a source of fuel – what could be better when you are trying to lose weight?

BARLEY

GI 25 (pearl)

One of the oldest cultivated cereals, barley is nutritious and high in soluble fibre, which helps to reduce the post-meal rise in blood glucose – it lowers the overall GI of a meal. In fact barley has one of the lowest GI values of any food. Look for products such as pearl barley to use in place of rice as a side dish, in porridge or to add to soups, stews and pilafs. You can also use barley as a substitute for rice to make risotto. Barley flakes, or rolled barley,

Wholegrains on the side

Try barley, buckwheat, bulghur or quinoa as a change from rice — vegetarian or wholefood cookbooks will give you some tasty recipes.

which have a light, nutty flavour, can be cooked as a cereal and used in baked goods and stuffing.

Serving suggestion

To make a zesty and satisfying chunky lentil and barley soup, cook a finely chopped onion gently in a little olive oil for about 10 minutes, or until soft and golden. Add 2 crushed cloves of garlic, ½ teaspoon of turmeric, 2 teaspoons of curry powder, ½ teaspoon of ground cumin and a teaspoon of minced chilli (or to taste) then add 1 litre (32 fl oz) of chicken stock or water. Stir in 110 grams (3 ¾ oz) of pearl barley, 100 grams (3½ oz) of red lentils and a 400 gram (14 oz) can of tomatoes. Bring to the boil, cover and simmer for about 45 minutes or until the lentils and barley are tender. Season to taste and serve sprinkled with chopped fresh parsley or coriander. Serves 4.

What's the difference?

❑ *Wholegrain foods* contain the whole grain – the bran, germ and endosperm. Even when processed much of the grain is intact – 'whole' or 'cracked'. It's these grainy bits that slow down the rate of digestion. A rule of thumb: if you can't see the grains then it's probably not low GI.

❑ *Wholemeal foods* contain all the components of the grain, but they have been milled to a finer texture and we digest them faster. Wholemeal foods usually have the same GI as their white counterparts. For example, white bread's GI is 70, wholemeal's is 71. Wholemeal foods are an important source of fibre and nutrients in a balanced diet.

BUCKWHEAT

GI 54

Gluten-free buckwheat is not a type of wheat or a true cereal at all – it's a herbaceous plant that produces triangular seeds. However, because the seeds are used in exactly the same way as cereal grains, that's what people think they are. Buckwheat has a rather nutty flavour and is a good source of protein, B vitamins, magnesium, potassium and soluble fibre.

It is easy to cook and you can use it in place of rice or other wholegrain cereals such as bulghur or add it to soups, stews and casseroles. Buckwheat flour is widely used for making pancakes, muffins, biscuits, and is an indispensable ingredient for Russia's blini and Japan's soba noodles.

Serving suggestion

To make buckwheat and buttermilk pancakes with berries, combine 130 grams (4½ oz) buckwheat flour, 35 grams (1¼ oz) wholemeal flour, 1½ teaspoons baking powder and 2 tablespoons of raw (demerara) sugar in a mixing bowl. Make a well in the centre and pour in 2 lightly beaten eggs, 250 ml (9 fl oz) buttermilk and 1 teaspoon of vanilla essence and whisk until smooth. Add a little more milk if the pancake batter is too thick. Heat a frypan over medium heat and lightly spray with olive oil. Pour 60 ml (2 fl oz) of the mixture into the pan and cook for 1–2 minutes each side, or until the pancakes are golden and cooked. Repeat with the remaining mixture. Top the pancakes with a spoonful of yoghurt and some blueberries. Serves 4 – two pancakes per person.

BULGHUR

GI 48

Also known as cracked wheat, bulghur is made from whole wheat grains that have been hulled and steamed before

grinding to crack the grain. The wheat grain remains virtually intact – it is simply cracked – and the wheat germ
and bran are retained, which preserves nutrients and
lowers the GI. With its wheaty flavour you can use bulghur
instead of rice or other grains in a range of recipes. Use
it as a breakfast cereal, in tabbouleh, or add it to pilafs,
vegetable burgers, stuffing, stews, salads and soups.

Serving suggestions

- Try this super-nutritious, high fibre mushroom and
  bulghur salad. Make a marinade with 3 tablespoons of
  lemon juice, 3 tablespoons of olive oil, a crushed garlic
  clove and a tablespoon each of freshly chopped parsley
  and mint (or more if you like). Marinate 125 grams (4½
  oz) of sliced button mushrooms and 2 chopped spring
  onions in the mixture for about an hour. Place 200 grams
  (7 oz) of bulghur in a bowl, cover with hot water and
  let it stand for about 20–30 minutes until the water is
  absorbed and the bulghur softens. Drain well, squeezing
  out excess water. Toss the bulghur with the marinated
  mushrooms and spoon into a serving dish. Serves 4.
- To make tabbouleh, cover 90 grams (3 oz) of bulghur
  with hot water and soak for 20–30 minutes to soften.
  Drain well and squeeze out the excess water. Add
  4 tablespoons finely chopped flat leaf parsley, 3 or
  4 chopped spring onions, 2 tablespoons of chopped
  mint and a chopped tomato. Stir in a dressing made
  with 2 tablespoons each of lemon juice and olive oil.
  Tabbouleh is best made ahead of serving time to let the
  flavours develop. Serves 4.
- Pilaf made with bulghur has a far lower GI than rice pilaf.
  Serve it with casseroles or as a meal on its own with
  chopped vegetables. Sauté a thinly sliced brown onion in
  1½ tablespoons of olive oil until it is translucent. Add a
  handful of crushed dry egg noodle vermicelli and stir

until it is pale gold in colour. Add 90 grams (3 oz) of bulghur and 250 ml (9 fl oz) of hot chicken stock. Cover and simmer on low heat for about 7 minutes or until it looks dry. Cover and stand for 10 minutes before serving. Serves 4 as a side dish.

QUINOA
GI 51

Quinoa (pronounced keen-wah) is a small, round, quick-cooking grain somewhat similar in colour to sesame seeds. It's a nutritional powerpack – an excellent source of low GI carbs, fibre and protein, and rich in B vitamins and minerals including iron, phosphorus, magnesium and zinc. You can also buy quinoa flakes and quinoa flour, but the GI of these products has not yet been published.

Health and organic food stores and larger super-markets are the best places to shop for quinoa. You may find it's a little more expensive than other grains. The wholegrain cooks in about 10–15 minutes and has a light, chewy texture and slightly nutty flavour and can be used as a substitute for many other grains. It is important to rinse quinoa thoroughly before cooking – the grains have a bitter-tasting coating designed by nature to discourage hungry hordes of birds.

Serving suggestion

- Make the most of this super grain – substitute gluten-free quinoa for rice, couscous, cracked wheat or barley in soups, stuffed vegetables, salads, stews and even in 'rice' pudding.
- To serve as a side dish, thoroughly rinse 1 cup of quinoa (if not pre-washed). Drain, place the grains in a medium-sized pot with 2 cups of water and bring to the boil. Reduce to a simmer, cover and leave to cook until all the water is absorbed.

- If you want a richer flavour, toast quinoa (but don't let it burn) in a dry pan for a few minutes before cooking as above.
- Give your day a hearty start with quinoa 'porridge' by adding 1 small apple, finely sliced, and a couple of tablespoons of sultanas to the pot while the quinoa is simmering. Add ½ teaspoon of cinnamon for extra flavour if you like. Serve with low fat milk and sweeten with honey or sugar to taste.

RYE
GI 34
Whole kernel rye is used to make bread, including pumpernickel and some crispbreads. It's an excellent source of fibre and also a good source of vitamins and minerals. It is more usually sold as rye flakes, which are the hulled, steamed and rolled rye grains. Like rolled oats, you can eat the flakes as a porridge or sprinkle them over bread before you bake it.

Serving suggestion
To make spicy stuffed tomatoes, gently cook 1 chopped onion in 1 tablespoon of olive oil for a minute or two. Add 2 crushed cloves of garlic and continue cooking until the onion is soft and golden. Add 1 diced medium-sized aubergine, 90 grams (3 oz) of rye flakes, 250 ml (9 fl oz) of water and 1 tablespoon of curry powder (or to taste). Stir, cover and simmer about 30 minutes or until the aubergine and rye flakes are tender and water is absorbed. Cut the tops off 4 large tomatoes and scoop out the insides; set the 'cups' aside. Chop the remaining tomato and add to the curry mixture. Remove the mixture from the heat and stir in a 150 gram (5½ oz) pot of plain low fat yoghurt and season with salt and freshly ground black pepper to taste. Spoon the curry mixture into the tomato cups and serve.

SEMOLINA

GI 55 (cooked)

Semolina is the coarsely milled inner part of the wheat grain called the endosperm. It is granular in appearance. The large particle size of semolina flour (compared with fine wheat flour) limits the swelling of its starch particles when cooked, which results in slower digestion, slower release of glucose into the blood stream and a lower GI.

You'll find durum wheat semolina in most supermarkets. You can use it to make homemade pasta or gnocchi or simply cook it and eat it as a hot cereal or make it into a traditional milk pudding. Use semolina to thicken sauces and gravies instead of plain flour.

Serving suggestion

To make semolina porridge, mix about 1 tablespoon of semolina with 3 tablespoons of low fat milk or water into a smooth paste. Slowly stir in 200 ml (7 fl oz) of semi-skimmed milk. Cook over a low heat, stirring continually for about 10 minutes to the desired consistency. Sweeten with a little honey or maple syrup, or serve with chopped fresh or canned fruit.

WHOLE WHEAT KERNELS

GI 41

As the most important cereal crop in the world, wheat – mainly in the form of bread and noodles – nourishes more people than any other grain. The bulk of the world's wheat is milled into flour – usually white flour. But there are forms of wheat, with their bran and germ intact, that can be eaten as a main or side dish. Whole wheat kernels (also called 'groats' or wheat berries) are a highly nutritious food, packed with B vitamins, protein and minerals including iron, magnesium and manganese. Think of them as the wheat version of rice – but allow for much longer cooking times. They have a strong, nutty flavour. Add them to hearty soups and stews, or use them when baking bread.

Couscous

Semolina is also used to make couscous (GI 65), a coarsely ground semolina pasta that's quick and easy to prepare. With a GI in the medium range, we suggest you enjoy this convenient food in moderation. Alternatively, adding low GI pulses such as chickpeas to couscous recipes is not only delicious, it reduces the overall GI of the dish. For a change, why not try barley couscous?

Serving suggestion

To cook whole kernel wheat, wash 200 grams (7 oz) of wheat then soak in 500 ml (17 fl oz) of water overnight. Place the rehydrated wheat in a pan with a little extra water if necessary and bring to the boil. Turn down the heat and simmer gently for about an hour until soft and the water is mostly absorbed. The cooked wheat will keep in a covered container in the refrigerator for about two weeks. Prepared this way, whole wheat kernels can be used for many dishes such as pilafs, tabbouleh, to bulk up meat dishes, and side dish substitutes for rice or noodles.

PULSES, INCLUDING BEANS, PEAS & LENTILS

For a low GI food that's easy on the budget, versatile, filling, low in calories and nutritious, look no further than pulses – beans, chickpeas and lentils.

Humans have long known about the benefits of eating pulses. Not only do they keep in the cupboard for a year or more, they are an excellent source of protein, easy to prepare and cost very little. When you cook them, they more than double in weight – 200 grams (7 oz) of dry beans makes 500 grams (1 lb 2 oz) of cooked beans – and when you eat them, you'll feel satisfied for longer.

So, what are they? Also known as legumes, pulses are the edible dried seeds found inside the mature pods of leguminous plants. Pulses include various types of beans, peas, chickpeas and lentils. Green peas are pulses but we most often eat them fresh as a green vegetable, so we have included them in the vegetable section. Peanuts are pulses, too, but since they are usually thought of as nuts we have included them in that section.

Whether you buy them dried, or opt for canned

convenience, you are choosing one of nature's lowest GI foods. They are high in fibre and packed with nutrients, providing protein, carbohydrate, B vitamins, folate and minerals. When you add pulses to meals and snacks, you reduce the overall GI of your diet because your body digests them slowly. This is primarily because their starch breaks down relatively slowly (or incompletely) during cooking and they contain tannins and enzyme inhibitors that also slow digestion.

Although they have an excellent shelf life, old beans take longer to cook than young, which is why it's a good idea to buy them from shops where you know turnover is brisk. Once home, store them in airtight containers in a cool, dry place – they will keep their colour better.

What about wind?

Pulses of all sorts, including baked beans, are renowned for producing flatulence (gas) and many jokes. The components responsible are indigestible sugars called raffinose, stachyose and verbascose that reach the large bowel intact where they are fermented by resident flora. Believe it or not, this is good for colonic health, increasing the proportion of good bifidobacteria and reducing potential pathogens. However, not all pulses will make you windy, and not everyone has the problem to the same extent. If you are worried about the social implications, cooking pulses in fresh water (not the water you soaked them in) reduces the problem, as does eating small amounts regularly – your body becomes used to them. Alternatively, to prevent the problem, add a minute amount of powdered asafoetida spice to the pot during cooking – no more than a quarter of a teaspoon per cup of dried beans or lentils. We have also been told that adding a teaspoon of powdered gelatine to the pot during cooking will help – but we haven't tried this one ourselves.

Canned bean convenience

Don't feel guilty about using canned beans – the main aim is to enjoy these low GI superfoods. The only disadvantage with canned beans is that they generally tend to be soft. If you like a firmer texture, especially in salads, you'll probably need to cook your own.

How much?

Pulses are an important part of a low GI diet which is why it's a good idea to try to include them in your meals at least twice a week as a starchy vegetable alternative – more often if you are vegetarian. One serving is equivalent to 100 grams (3½ oz) of cooked beans, lentils, chickpeas or whole dried or split peas.

Serving suggestions

You can substitute one 400 gram (14 oz) can of beans for 150 grams (5½ oz) of dried beans.

- Drain and rinse canned beans and add them directly to soups, stews, salads or curries.
- Top lettuce with kidney beans or chickpeas marinated in an oil and vinegar dressing.
- Add beans or chickpeas to vegetable soups or minestrone.
- Make a puréed bean dip and serve with carrot or celery sticks, blanched mangetouts or cucumber strips.
- Create your own bean filling for tacos and burritos by mashing canned chilli beans with a fork.
- Purée cooked yellow split peas or canned navy beans to use as a base for soups or chowders.

Preparing dried pulses

1. **Wash** Wash thoroughly in a colander or sieve first, keeping an eye out for any small stones or 'foreign' material (especially with lentils).
2. **Soak** Soaking plumps the beans, makes them softer and tastier and reduces cooking times a little. Place them in a saucepan, cover with about three times their volume of cold water and soak overnight or for at least four hours. As a rule of thumb, the larger the seed, the longer the soaking time required. There's no need to soak lentils or split peas.
3. **Cook** Drain, rinse thoroughly, then add fresh water – two to three times the volume of the pulses. Bring to the boil then reduce the heat and simmer until tender. Generally, you will need to simmer lentils and peas for 45–60 minutes and beans and chickpeas for 1–2 hours, but check the recipe instructions. A couple of points to keep in mind:

❑ Adding salt to the water during cooking will slow down water absorption and the pulses will take longer to cook.
❑ Make sure that pulses are tender before you add acidic flavourings such as lemon juice or tomatoes. Once they are in an acid medium they won't get any softer no matter how long you cook them.

Time-saving tips

❑ If you don't have time to soak pulses overnight, add three times the volume of water to rinsed beans, bring to the boil for a few minutes then remove from the heat and soak for an hour. Drain, rinse, add fresh water then cook as usual.
❑ Cooked pulses freeze well. Prepare a large quantity of beans or chickpeas and freeze in meal-sized batches to use as required.
❑ Store soaked or cooked beans in an airtight container in the fridge. They will keep for several days.

Where to buy beans?

These days supermarkets stock a wide range of dried and canned beans. For the more unusual beans, check out your local health food store or Greek, Turkish, Middle Eastern, South American or kosher delicatessen or produce market.

BAKED BEANS
GI 48 (canned in tomato sauce)

Baked beans are a popular ready-to-eat form of pulse, an easy way to introduce children to the world of beans, and available in convenient single-serve cans. Haricot (navy) beans are most commonly used for baked beans. If you make your own baked bean recipe, it will have a lower GI.

Serving suggestions

- Top half a jacket potato cooked in the microwave with a scoop or two of canned or homemade baked beans sprinkled with a little grated cheese.
- A scoop or two of baked beans is a healthy addition to any meal or a satisfying breakfast or light meal served on grainy toast.

BLACK BEANS
GI 30 (home-cooked)

The black bean or black kidney bean is the small, shiny bean with an earthy sweet flavour often used in South and Central American and Caribbean cooking, and Mexican dishes such as refried beans. Add them to chilli con carne or to bean soups and salads for extra flavour and texture. In Latin-American-style dishes, a spicy bean mix made with black or red kidney beans is often served over rice.

Serving suggestion

Use leftover chicken and rice to make these tasty burritos. Preheat the oven to 180°C (350°F, Gas mark 4). Wrap 6 large tortillas in foil and warm in the oven. Cook 1 chopped onion and 1 crushed clove of garlic in a tablespoon of vegetable oil, stirring occasionally until softened. Add 200 grams (7 oz) of chopped cooked chicken, 200 grams (7 oz) of cooked or canned black beans, 200 grams (7 oz) of cooked basmati rice and 1 can of diced tomatoes. To serve, spoon about 3–4 heaped tablespoons of the filling into the centre of the warmed tortilla. Sprinkle 1 tablespoon of grated low fat cheese on top, fold in the ends, then roll the tortilla around the filling. Place in a large shallow baking dish. Sprinkle 100 grams (3½ oz) cup of grated low fat cheese on top of burritos, then cover with foil and heat in the oven for about 10 minutes, or until the cheese is melted and the filling is hot. Serve topped with chopped coriander. Makes 6.

BLACK-EYED BEANS
GI 42

Also known as cowpeas, Southern peas and black-eyed peas, these beans are medium-sized, kidney-shaped and cream-coloured with a distinctive black 'eye' and a subtle flavour. They are a popular 'soul food' in the southern states of the US where they are traditionally served with pork. Add black-eyed beans to soups and stews or serve as a side dish.

Serving suggestions

- Cook chopped leeks, onions and carrots with crushed garlic in a little olive oil. Add cooked or canned black-eyed, kidney and borlotti beans, canned tomatoes plus fresh thyme and bay leaves and a chopped red chilli to make a Mediterranean-style vegetable casserole.
- Soak a cup of black-eyed beans overnight then simmer in fresh water for about 30 minutes until tender. Drain and cool, then add chopped tomato and celery. Toss with a dressing of 2 tablespoons chopped parsley, 1 tablespoon seeded mustard, 1 crushed clove of garlic and 3 tablespoons each of olive oil and wine vinegar.

BORLOTTI BEANS
GI 41 (canned)

This medium-sized bean has a creamy texture, slightly nutty flavour and reddish-black to magenta streaks that fade to brown during cooking. It is widely used for soups, stews, casseroles and in salads and the delicious pasta and bean soup you will find served all over Italy (although they tend to use cannellini beans in the south).

Serving suggestions

- Combine a cup of cooked beans with 2–3 tablespoons of semi-dried tomatoes and a handful of baby spinach leaves in a balsamic dressing.
- Add borlotti beans to a salad of tuna chunks, onion rings, tomato slices, olives and chopped fresh parsley.
- Mash cooked or canned borlotti beans with sweet potato, 125 ml (4 fl oz) of heated semi-skimmed milk and some freshly grated nutmeg. Leave some of the beans whole for texture.

BUTTER BEANS
GI 31 (home cooked)
GI 36 (canned)

Sometimes called large lima beans, butter beans are a flat-shaped white bean with a smooth, creamy, slightly sweet flavour. Add to soups, stews and salads or simply heat and serve as a side dish topped with finely chopped fresh herbs.

Serving suggestions

- Add a cup of cooked butter beans and a crushed clove of garlic to steamed sweet potato (or yam) and mash as usual. Season to taste with a little salt and freshly ground black pepper and add enough water or low fat milk or soya milk for a creamy consistency.

- Dip pitta crisps into a butter bean purée. Purée a drained can of butter beans (or any white bean) with a crushed clove of garlic in the food processor slowly, pouring in just enough oil and lemon juice to create the desired consistency.

CANNELLINI BEANS
GI 31 (canned)

Also known as white kidney beans, cannellini beans are large, smooth-textured, mild-flavoured, kidney-shaped beans with a creamy white skin. They are used in soups, salads, stews, casseroles, bean pots such as the French cassoulet and in many Italian dishes.

Serving suggestions

- Add cannellini beans to puréed vegetable soups for a creamy texture. Simmer cauliflower florets until tender in chicken stock then blend with a cup of cooked beans and season to taste with salt and freshly ground black pepper. Top with freshly grated nutmeg and finely chopped parsley and serve.
- Make a salad of cannellini beans and finely sliced fennel tossed in a tangy lemon, oil and vinegar dressing and top with finely chopped flat leaf parsley.

CHICKPEAS
GI 28 (home cooked)
GI 40 (canned)

Also known as garbanzo beans or ceci, these versatile caramel-coloured pulses have a nutty flavour and firm texture. Popular in Middle Eastern, Mediterranean and Mexican cooking, they are the main ingredient in special-ties such as hummous and felafel and the basis for many vegetarian dishes. Keep a can in the cupboard or cooked chickpeas in the refrigerator and add them to soups, stews and salads or to a tomato-based sauce served with couscous or rice. After soaking, whole chickpeas can be roasted with salt and spices to make a crunchy low GI snack that's every bit as more-ish as crisps!

Serving suggestions

- Combine 2 oranges separated into segments, a drained and rinsed 400 gram (14 oz) can of chickpeas and a finely sliced fennel bulb (or two if small ones). Toss in a dressing made with olive oil, vinegar and orange juice for a tangy salad.
- To make a spicy pilaf, simmer a finely chopped onion in a little olive oil until soft, then add a cup of chopped button mushrooms and a crushed clove of garlic. Stir in 150 grams (5½ oz) of basmati rice, a teaspoon of garam masala and a cup of cooked chickpeas. Pour over 375 ml (13 fl oz) of chicken stock, bring to the boil then reduce the heat to very low, cover and simmer gently for 10–12 minutes or until the rice is tender and all the liquid is absorbed.

CANNED MIXED BEANS
GI 37 (canned)

Canned bean mixes which include red kidney beans, chickpeas and lima and butter beans make it easy to add protein and boost flavour and fibre to meals including soups and stews. You can also add canned mixed beans to your salad wraps, sandwiches and rolls for a lunch that lasts.

Serving suggestions

- For a meal in minutes, combine drained and rinsed mixed beans with baby spinach leaves, chopped spring onions, cucumber, yellow pepper, sliced radishes, finely sliced celery and halved or quartered cherry tomatoes and toss in a light lemony oil and vinegar dressing.
- Boost the flavour and fibre of a home-made tomato soup by adding a can of drained, rinsed four bean mix.

HARICOT BEANS
GI 33 (home-cooked)
GI 38 (canned)
These small, white, oval-shaped beans, sometimes called navy beans, are the ones most often used in the manufacture of commercial baked beans. They have a mild flavour and combine well in soups and stews.

Serving suggestion
Make your own baked beans to serve for breakfast on grainy toast or as a side dish. Combine a small chopped onion, 2 small diced peppers (red or green) and 600 grams (1 lb 3 oz) of cooked or canned haricot beans in a large casserole dish. Add 4 tablespoons of pure floral honey, 2 tablespoons of Dijon mustard, 1 tablespoon of white wine vinegar, 125 ml (4 fl oz) of tomato sauce and a few twists of freshly ground black pepper. Mix well then cover and cook in a preheated oven (180°C, 350°F, Gas mark 4) for about 45 minutes to an hour. Serves 6–8 as a side dish.

HUMMOUS
GI 6 (regular)
Hummous – puréed chickpeas, lemon juice, tahini, olive oil, garlic and sometimes ingredients such as roasted red peppers – is one of the most popular foods to emerge from the Middle East. It can be served as part of a mezze platter or used as a dip with pitta bread, or raw or blanched vegetables such as carrot and celery sticks. It's widely available in the refrigerator section of supermarkets and fresh produce stores, in specialist delis, or as a takeaway from Lebanese or Turkish restaurants.

Serving suggestions
- Use hummous as a spread for sandwiches, as a topping on grilled fish, chicken, with baked potatoes, or in a wrap with kebabs and salad or a falafel roll.

- To make your own, combine a 400 gram (14 oz) can of chickpeas (drained, reserving the liquid), 135 grams (4½ oz) of tahini (sesame seed paste), a large clove of garlic, chopped, 80 ml (2½ fl oz) lemon juice, plus a little salt and freshly ground black pepper to taste. Process in a blender or food processor, adding enough of the reserved chickpea liquid to make a smooth consistency.

LENTILS
GI 26 (red, home cooked)
GI 30 (green, home cooked)
GI 48 (green, canned)

Lentils are one food that people with diabetes should learn to love – they can eat them until the cows come home. In fact, we have found that no matter how much of them people eat, they have only a small effect on blood glucose levels. They are one of nature's superfoods – rich in protein, fibre and B vitamins and often used as substitutes for meat in vegetarian recipes.

All colours and types of lentils have a similar low GI value, which is increased slightly if you opt to buy them canned and add them towards the end of cooking time. Lentils have a fairly bland, earthy flavour that combines well with onions, garlic and spices. They cook quickly to a soft consistency and are used to make Indian dhal, a spiced lentil purée. Lentils also thicken any kind of soup or extend meat casseroles.

Serving suggestions

- Make a meal of lentil soup and low GI bread – you will feel completely satisfied. Canned lentil soup (GI 44) is a convenient, quick meal when you don't have time to prepare your own.
- To make a vegetarian lentil burger, simmer a chopped onion in olive oil for a few minutes to soften. In a bowl

thoroughly combine 400 grams (14 oz) of canned and drained lentils with the onion mix and 400 grams (14 oz) of mashed potato or sweet potato, season to taste with salt and freshly ground black pepper, adding a dash of Tabasco or chilli sauce for flavour. Form into patties and cook them on both sides until browned in the oven, on the barbecue or in a pan and combine with salad, tomato slices, chutney and grainy rolls.

- For an easy alternative to mashed potato, bring to the boil 250 ml (9 fl oz) of chicken or vegetable stock, 150 grams (5½ oz) of split red lentils and 1 bay leaf, then simmer until the lentils are mushy and thick. Season with salt and freshly ground black pepper. You may also like to add a teaspoon of curry powder for extra flavour.

LIMA BEANS

GI 32 (baby frozen)

The lima bean, a larger variety of the butter bean, comes from Peru. Baby lima beans, also called sieva beans, cook faster. They are popular in the US where they are served as a vegetable side dish. Dried and canned lima beans have a buttery flavour and are used in soups, stews and salads. If you are cooking your own, bring them to the boil slowly to prevent the skin from slipping off.

Serving suggestions

- Toss a cup of cooked beans with 3–4 tablespoons of sun-dried tomatoes, 30 grams (1 oz) of sultanas and 30 grams (1 oz) of chopped pecan nuts in a dressing made with the juice of a lemon and 2 tablespoons of olive oil. Season to taste and serve with finely chopped fresh dill.
- Gently warm 200 grams (7 oz) of cooked or canned lima beans in a pan with 60 ml (2 fl oz) of freshly squeezed lemon juice, a tablespoon of olive oil, 2 finely

chopped cloves of garlic and 2 teaspoons of fresh thyme (leaves picked) until just heated through. Toss in a salad bowl with 8 cooked baby beetroot cut into quarters, and a handful each of rocket and baby spinach leaves. Top with crumbled feta and serve.

Marrowfat or 'mushy' peas

Marrowfat peas (GI 39) are a completely different variety from the green or garden pea. They are large yellow peas that, like all pulses, are rich in nutrients and have a low GI. The maro pea was introduced to the UK from Japan over 100 years ago because the climate was suitable for pea growing. It then became known as 'marrowfat' because of its plump shape. You can buy marrowfat peas dried, in cans or as canned 'mushy peas'. They make delicious pea soup.

MUNG BEANS
GI 39 (home cooked)

Also known as green gram or golden gram, dried mung beans are small, olive-green beans that are used in many Asian cuisines for savoury dishes such as India's green gram dhal or to make a paste for popular sweets. The starch from mung beans is used in making bean thread and cellophane noodles. Like all pulses, they are a good source of fibre, iron and protein. You can buy sprouted mung beans in punnets – a useful source of vitamin C.

Serving suggestions

- Add mung bean sprouts as an extra vegetable to a stir-fry or fried rice at the end of cooking.
- Combine 100 grams (3½ oz) of mung bean sprouts, 100 grams (3½ oz) of baby spinach, 100 grams (3½ oz)

of baby rocket, 1 sliced cucumber, 1 punnet of baby tomatoes, halved, ½ an avocado, sliced, 1 small finely sliced red onion and 100 grams (3½ oz) of pitted black olives in a large salad bowl with a dressing made from olive oil, balsamic vinegar and a dash of lemon juice. Serves 4.

PEANUTS
See page 200

PEAS
GI 22 (whole dried, home cooked)
GI 32 (yellow or green split peas)
Like other pulses, dried peas are a nutritional storehouse and because they are slowly digested, a little goes a long way. Whole dried or blue peas are the dried version of garden peas and traditionally used in English dishes such as 'pease pudding' and mushy peas. Soak them before cooking.

Yellow or green split peas come from a variety of garden pea with the husk removed. They tend to disintegrate and are traditionally used for pea and ham soup and yellow split peas for making Indian dhal.

Serving suggestions

- Your local Indian takeaway will sell prepared dhals. Combined with flat bread and basmati rice, dhal makes a delicious low GI light vegetarian meal. To make your own dhal, rinse and drain 200 grams (7 oz) of red lentils and place in a saucepan with ½ a teaspoon of turmeric and a pinch of chilli powder. Add 375 ml (13 fl oz) of boiling water and cook for 15 minutes or until the lentils are very soft, but still retain their shape. Season to taste with salt. Heat 1 tablespoon of margarine or olive oil in a small frypan and gently cook a small finely chopped onion until soft and golden – about

> ### Dhal (or dal)
>
> Dhal can refer to dried pulses (Bengal gram, split peas, channa and lentils) as well as the purée that's usually served with Indian meals.

10 minutes. Stir 1 teaspoon of garam masala into the onion mixture, stir briskly for 30 seconds, then add 1 teaspoon of coriander and combine with the lentils. Season to taste with salt and freshly ground black pepper. You may also like to add a squeeze of lime.
- Make a thick pea soup with 350 grams (12 oz) of split peas, 2 finely chopped onions, 2 finely chopped carrots, 2 finely sliced sticks of celery and 2 litres (3½ pints) of stock or water. Add a bay leaf for flavouring, season with freshly ground black pepper and, for extra oomph, add a bacon bone or two while the soup is cooking.

See also Green peas, page 134.

PINTO BEANS
GI 39 (home-cooked)
GI 45 (canned)
This medium-sized mottled bean ('pinto' means painted) turns pinkish-brown when cooked. It's a staple in Latin-American cooking and used whole or made into refried beans as a filling for burritos or tacos.

Serving suggestion

- Make a colourful and crunchy bean mix for tacos. Combine 2 cups of cooked pinto beans with a finely diced green pepper, a cup of juicy red chopped tomatoes, 2 sliced spring onions, 1 cup of sweetcorn kernels (straight off the cob is best), ½ teaspoon of ground cumin and salt and freshly ground black pepper to taste. Serve with tacos and bowls of guacamole, shredded lettuce and grated low fat cheese. Serves 4.
- To make refried beans, heat a little olive or sesame oil in a frypan over medium heat. Add 1 finely sliced onion and 2 cloves of crushed garlic and cook very gently until soft and golden (about 10 minutes). Stir in 2 cups of cooked pinto (or black) beans, 2 teaspoons of cumin

and 125 ml (4 fl oz) of water or vegetable stock. Mash the beans into the liquid, adding more stock if the mixture seems too dry. Season to taste with salt and freshly ground black pepper.

RED KIDNEY BEANS
GI 36 (canned)
These tasty red beans are a popular addition to vegetarian and meat chilli dishes and nachos, tacos and burritos. Not only do red kidney beans play a leading role in Mexican and 'Tex-Mex' cuisines, a scoop is a sustaining side dish with main meals and adds substance to soups, stews and salads.

Serving suggestions

- Stir into a homemade or bought tangy tomato salsa to add a Mexican flavour.
- Create a colourful bean salad by combining a 400 gram (14 oz) can of kidney beans (drained) in a serving bowl with 200 grams (7 oz) each of cooked green beans and cooked yellow beans sliced on the diagonal. Finely slice half a red pepper, half a green pepper and 2 stalks of celery. Toss the beans and vegetables in a light dressing made with balsamic vinegar and olive oil. Coat the salad well – you will need about 125 ml (4 fl oz) of dressing. Serves 4–6 as a side dish.

ROMANO BEANS
GI 46 (home-cooked)
Sometimes referred to as Italian flat beans, romano beans can be eaten as a snap bean when very young or as a dried bean during later stages of maturity. They are used in a wide variety of bean and chilli dishes, soups and salads.

Tofu

Tofu has little or no carbs. It's a cheese-like curd made from soyabeans, and although it is not high in fibre, it's a low-cost, high-protein, low fat bean food that will surprise you with its versatility. By itself, tofu is bland, so marinate it in soy sauce, ginger, chilli and garlic or try it as part of a well-seasoned dish such as a stir-fry.

Serving suggestion

To make a spinach and bean stir-fry, gently cook 2 chopped spring onions and a finely chopped clove of garlic in a little olive oil. Add a seeded and diced red pepper and toss to heat through for 2–3 minutes. Stir in 150 grams (5½ oz) of baby spinach leaves, 2 tablespoons of chopped fresh chives and 400 grams (14 oz) of cooked romano beans. When heated through, season to taste, and serve topped with freshly grated nutmeg alongside bulghur, quinoa or low GI rice. Serves 4.

SOYABEANS
GI 14 (canned)
GI 18 (home cooked)

Soyabeans and soya products are the nutritional power-house of the pulse family. They have been a staple part of Asian diets for thousands of years and are an excellent source of protein. They're also rich in fibre, iron, zinc and vitamin B. They are lower in carbohydrate and higher in fat than other pulses, but the majority of the fat is polyunsaturated. Soyabeans are a rich source of phytochemicals, especially phytoestrogens, and have been linked with improvements in blood cholesterol levels, relief from menopausal symptoms and lower rates of cancer in many studies.

Serving suggestions

- Use canned soyabeans in place of other beans in any recipe.
- Make a quick soyabean and vegetable curry with chopped onions, garlic, carrots, tomatoes, cauliflower and broccoli using vegetable stock and your favourite curry paste.

NUTS

People who eat nuts once a week have less heart disease than those who don't eat any nuts. There are probably several reasons. Nuts contain a variety of anti-oxidants, which keep blood vessels healthy; arginine, an amino acid that helps keep blood flowing smoothly; folate; and fibre, which can both lower cholesterol levels. Although nuts are high in fat (averaging around 50 per cent), it is largely unsaturated, so they make a healthy substitute for foods such as biscuits, cakes, crisps, pastries and chocolate. They also contain relatively little carbohydrate, so most do not have a GI value.

How do you halve your risk of developing heart disease? By eating a small handful of nuts five to seven times a week!

Nuts are one of the richest sources of vitamin E, with a small handful of mixed nuts providing more than 20 per cent of the recommended daily intake. The vitamin E content may explain the findings from a recent study from Harvard University School of Public Health which found that increased nut consumption, including natural peanut butter, may improve the body's ability to balance glucose and insulin.

How much?

One serving provides 10 grams of fat and is equivalent to:

- 15 grams (½ oz) – about 10 small or 5 large – nuts or a tablespoon of seeds
- 3 teaspoons (15 ml) peanut butter or Nutella®

How much a day?

Aim for a small handful (no fingers) of nuts most days.

- Smaller eaters: 1 serving most days
- Medium eaters: 1 serving a day
- Bigger eaters: 1–2 servings most days

Serving suggestions

- Use nuts and seeds in food preparation. Try toasted cashews in a chicken stir-fry; sprinkle walnuts over a pear and radicchio salad with a light blue cheese dressing; or top fruit desserts or muesli with natural almonds.
- Add toasted pine nuts to your favourite pasta dish.
- Sprinkle a mixture of chopped nuts and linseeds over cereal or salads, or add to baked goods such as muffins and slices.

CASHEWS

GI 22

Cashews, like all nuts, are cholesterol free and high in protein. Their carbohydrate content is quite low, which accounts for their low GI value. They do have a high fat content (almost half their total weight) but it is less than any other type of nut and three-quarters of it is heart-healthy polyunsaturated and monunsaturated fat. Cashews are also rich in several B vitamins and the minerals copper, magnesium and zinc. Because of their high nutrient content and energy density (calories/ kilojoules) you can eat cashews several times a week, but keep the amounts you eat small and look for unsalted varieties.

Serving suggestion

Cashews make a healthy addition to salads, rice dishes and desserts and are a popular ingredient in Asian stir-fries.

NUTELLA®

GI 33

Nutella® is a sweetened chocolate spread based on hazel-nuts, cocoa, skimmed milk powder and peanut oil and is a favourite even with non-chocoholics. About half its sugar content is milk sugar (lactose). Its fat content is high but the fats are mainly mono- and polyunsaturated (just like peanut butter), so it can be a healthy addition to the balanced diet of any active person.

Serving suggestions

- Add to banana smoothies, or stir a little through plain yoghurt for a chocolate fix.
- Soften a little Nutella® in the microwave and serve with a scoop of low fat ice-cream sprinkled with crunchy natural or toasted muesli.

PEANUTS

GI 14

A low carb but high fat, high protein food (50 per cent fat and 25 per cent protein), peanuts grow under the ground – they are also known as groundnuts. Technically a pulse, they are an excellent source of vitamins B and E and so low in carbohydrate that their GI doesn't really count – although their fat content does! Because peanuts are such a tasty and convenient finger food they are easily overeaten, so give yourself a specific ration. And stick to it!

All processed peanuts are quality-controlled for the presence of fungus that produces a toxin called aflatoxin, one of the most carcinogenic substances known. Because peanuts in the shell are not screened, throw away any mouldy ones. And a word to the wise: choose dry roasted peanuts and avoid salt.

Peanut allergy is an increasingly common food allergy especially in children. It occurs in approximately 1 in 50 children and 1 in 200 adults and is the allergy most likely to cause anaphylaxis (which involves swelling in the gut, respiratory tract and/or cardiovascular system) and death. Symptoms of allergy include itching, especially around the mouth, swelling tongue, flushed face, cramping, difficulty breathing, diarrhoea and vomiting. If peanut allergy is suspected urgent medical attention should be sought. One-third of all peanut-allergic people are also allergic to tree nuts such as brazil nuts, hazelnuts, walnuts, almonds, macadamia nuts, pistachios, pecans, pine nuts and cashews.

Serving suggestions

- Make up trail mixes with peanuts, sultanas, dried fruit and sunflower seeds for a no-fuss snack on the run.
- Sprinkle crushed nuts over salads for flavour and crunch or stir crushed nuts and chopped dried fruit through low fat yoghurt.
- Add crushed peanuts to the mix when baking biscuits or slices.

PEANUT BUTTER
GI 14

This delicious treat is made from ground nuts. The healthiest type of peanut butter has no added salt and is made from fresh, unroasted peanuts. Peanut butter is an excellent source of niacin and a good source of magnesium. The best way to include more peanut butter in your diet is to use it in place of butter or margarine.

Serving suggestions

- Top toast with peanut butter and banana or grated apple.
- Make a salad sandwich with lettuce, tomato, grated carrot, sprouts and cucumber, using peanut butter as the spread.
- Use peanut butter to make a satay sauce and serve with vegetables and kebabs.

FISH & SEAFOOD

We can't measure a GI for fish because it doesn't contain any carbohydrate. However, it is an important part of a balanced diet and we now know that just one serve of fish or seafood a week may reduce the risk of a fatal heart attack by about 40 per cent. The likely protective components of fish are the very long chain omega-3 fatty acids. Our bodies only make small amounts of these fatty acids which is why we rely on dietary sources, especially fish and seafood.

Increased fish consumption is linked to a reduced risk of coronary heart disease, improvements in mood, lower rates of depression, better blood fat levels and enhanced immunity.

How much?

Eat fish, including fresh, frozen, canned and smoked, one to three times a week as an alternative to a serve of meat, chicken or egg.

One serving is equivalent to:

- 150 grams (5½ oz) raw fish or seafood
- 115 grams (4 oz) grilled or steamed fish
- 100 grams (3½ oz) canned fish (drained)

Which fish?

Oily fish, which tend to have darker coloured flesh and a stronger fish flavour, are the richest source of omega-3 fats.

- Fresh fish with higher levels of omega-3s are: Atlantic salmon; smoked salmon; Atlantic, Pacific and Spanish mackerel; sea mullet; southern bluefin tuna; and swordfish. Eastern and Pacific oysters and squid (calamari) are also rich sources.
- Canned pink and red salmon (including the bones),

sardines, mackerel and, to a lesser extent, tuna, are all rich sources of omega-3s; look for canned fish packed in water, canola oil, olive oil, tomato sauce or brine, and drain well.

A WORD ABOUT FISH AND MERCURY

While there are many benefits of eating fish, if you are pregnant you do need to be careful about the types of fish you eat. Some fish contain high levels of mercury which can be harmful to your baby.

FSA (Food Standards Agency United Kingdom) recently revised their guidelines on mercury in fish. They advise that pregnant women, women planning pregnancy and children under 16 should continue to consume a variety of fish as part of a healthy diet but should avoid certain species – shark (flake), marlin and swordfish, and possibly limit the amount of tuna they eat. As an alternative to tuna enjoy other oily fish such as mackerel, herring, pilchards, sardines, trout and salmon.

For more information consult the website www. food.gov.uk

FISH FINGERS
GI 38

Fish fingers have a measurable GI because of their breadcrumb coating. Although low GI, they may be high in saturated fat, depending on the oil used in their manufacture. Check the food label carefully. Oven baking or grilling are the healthiest ways to cook them and, of course, serve them with plenty of vegetables or salad.

LEAN MEAT, CHICKEN & EGGS

As with fish and seafood, GI is not relevant to protein-rich meat, chicken and eggs. These foods are valuable inclusions in a healthy diet, however, not only for protein, but also for essential vitamins and minerals. Red meat is the best dietary source of iron, the nutrient used in carrying oxygen in our blood, and the main source of zinc, which is a part of over 100 enzymes throughout the body. Good iron and zinc status can improve your energy levels and exercise tolerance.

Lean meat, chicken and eggs are valuable additions to a healthy diet thanks to their protein, and nutrients such as iron, zinc, vitamin B12, niacin and other B vitamins.

A chronic shortage of iron leads to anaemia, with symptoms including pale skin, excessive tiredness, breathlessness and decreased attention span. Even mild iron deficiency can cause unexplained fatigue.

Although chicken contains about one-third as much iron as meat, it is readily absorbed, as it is from red meat, and provides a versatile, nutrient-rich alternative. Eggs also contain valuable amounts of the nutrients found in meat, although the iron is not as well absorbed. The cholesterol content of eggs is only a concern if you have high cholesterol levels and/or your total diet is high in saturated fat. Omega-3-enriched eggs, meat and chicken also make a significant contribution to long chain omega-3 fats which are so vital in human brain development and function.

How much?

Although nutritious, meat, chicken and eggs do not have to be a part of everyone's diet. After all, there are countless healthy vegetarians in the world! If you are not vegetarian, we suggest eating lean meat three times a week in addition to eggs or skinless chicken once or twice a week, accompanied by plenty of salad and vegetables. One serving is equivalent to:

- 100 grams (3½ oz) raw lean meat or chicken
- 2 medium eggs
- 1 small chop, fat removed
- 100 grams (3½ oz) cooked lean mince
- ½ skinless chicken breast
- 1 large chicken drumstick

How much a day?

One or two servings a day is appropriate for most people; bigger eaters may want a little more.

- Smaller eaters: 1–2 servings a day
- Medium eaters: 2–3 servings a day
- Bigger eaters: 3 servings a day

Shopping tips

- Choose lower fat meat products such as pastrami, leg ham and rolled turkey breast.
- Choose lean cuts of meat.
- Cut visible fat including skin from meat and poultry and drain away the fat after cooking.

Serving suggestions

- Marinate skinless chicken or lean meat to add flavour and moisture before grilling or baking. Try combinations of olive oil, red wine and garlic or lemon juice, olive oil, fresh herbs and pepper.
- Try cooking fresh fish in the microwave for a quick meal, basted with soy sauce, lemon juice or yoghurt and seasoned with fresh dill, paprika or curry spices. One fillet takes 60–90 seconds on full power.
- Pan-fry or stir-fry strips of lean meat or chicken in a

non-stick pan using small amounts of olive or rapeseed oil. Add flavour with ginger, garlic, chilli, lemon zest, adding sauces such as soy, oyster, hoi sin etc, after cooking.

• Enjoy poached eggs with grainy bread and baby spinach; scrambled eggs with salmon; or an omelette or frittata with lots of vegetables.

LOW FAT DAIRY FOODS & CALCIUM-ENRICHED SOYA PRODUCTS

Calcium is the most abundant mineral in our bodies. It builds our bones and teeth and is involved in muscle contraction and relaxation, blood clotting, nerve function and regulation of blood pressure. If we don't get enough calcium in our diet, our bodies will draw it out of our bones. Over a period of time, this can lead to osteoporosis, loss of height, curvature of the spine and periodontal disease (disease of the bones supporting our teeth).

The key to strong, healthy bones is making sure we have plenty of calcium in our diet. Low fat dairy foods are among the richest sources and, for most of us, the easiest way to get the calcium we need.

Studies are now showing that calcium:

• can help lower high blood pressure
• may protect against cancer, particularly cancer of the bladder, bowel and colon, and possibly against breast, ovarian, pancreas and skin cancers
• can favourably influence blood fat levels and reduce the risk of stroke
• can reduce the risk of kidney stones
• can assist in weight regulation

Dairy foods

Dairy foods are recommended throughout childhood and beyond. Not only are they an important source of calcium, but they also provide energy, protein, carbohydrate and vitamins A, B and D. Virtually all dairy foods have low GI values – largely thanks to lactose, the sugar found naturally in milk, which has a low GI of 46.

By choosing low fat varieties of milk, yoghurt, ice-cream and custard, you will enjoy a food that provides you with sustained energy, boosting your calcium intake but not your saturated fat intake. Although cheese is a good source of calcium, it is not a source of carbohydrate as its lactose is drawn off in the whey during production. This means that GI is not relevant to cheese.

What about lactose intolerance?

Lactose, the sugar in milk, is a disaccharide ('double sugar') that needs to be digested into its component sugars before our bodies can absorb it. The two sugars (glucose and galactose) compete with each other for absorption. Once absorbed, the galactose is mainly metabolised in the liver and produces very little effect on our blood glucose levels. The remaining sugar, glucose, is present in a small enough amount not to cause a spike in blood glucose.

Some people are lactose intolerant because the enzyme lactase is not active in their small intestine. Children who are lactose intolerant often outgrow this by five years of age. If you are lactose intolerant, you should still be able to enjoy cheese – which is virtually lactose free – and yoghurt. The micro-organisms in yoghurt are active in digesting lactose during passage through the small intestine. Alternatively, try lactose-reduced or lactose-free milk and milk products, or low GI, low fat, calcium-enriched non-dairy alternatives such as soya milk. Note that rice milk has a high GI value (GI 92).

Non-dairy calcium sources

If you eat only plant foods or want to avoid dairy products, you may turn to soya beverages, yoghurts and desserts as an alternative. Soya products are not naturally high in calcium so look for calcium-fortified products if you are relying on them as a source of calcium.

Other non-dairy options that will boost your calcium intake are foods such as almonds, Brazil nuts, sesame seeds, dried figs, dried apricots, soyabeans, Asian greens such as bok choi, fish with edible bones such as salmon and sardines, calcium-enriched tofu and calcium-fortified breakfast cereals.

How much?

One serving is equivalent to:

- 200 ml (7 fl oz) semi-skimmed milk
- 200 ml (7 fl oz) calcium-enriched low fat soya milk
- 150 grams (5½ oz) pot low fat yoghurt or calcium-enriched soya yoghurt
- 30 grams (1 oz) reduced fat hard cheese
- 200 ml (7 fl oz) low fat custard or 8 scoops (400 ml/ 14 fl oz) of low fat ice-cream are calcium-equivalent options but are higher in calories, so don't rely on them routinely.

How much a day?

Everyone should aim to eat or drink at least two or three servings of dairy foods or calcium-enriched soya products per day to meet calcium needs.

- Smaller eaters: 2 servings
- Medium eaters: 2 servings
- Bigger eaters: 3 servings

Boning up

We build our maximum bone strength by the time we reach about 20 years old. From our early 30s, bone calcium starts decreasing, but an adequate calcium intake, among other things, can help stop the decline.

Weight control

Recent research suggests that people who include more dairy foods in their diet are better able to control their weight. Calcium is required to burn fat but it's also possible that some components of dairy inhibit fat absorption.

Serving suggestions

The experts tell us that it only takes 21 days to start building a new health habit. Here are some simple ways to get started and make sure you get two or three servings of dairy foods each day.

- Start your day with a fruit smoothie.
- Top your breakfast cereal with yoghurt.
- Relax with a café latte mid-morning.
- Add a slice of cheese or a dollop of ricotta to your sandwich.
- Reach for a glass of cool milk for a refreshing snack.
- Follow your main meal with a dairy dessert.
- End the day with warm milk and honey to ensure a good night's sleep.

Did you know?

In Britain at least two and a half million young people and women do not eat enough calcium, the building block for strong bones and teeth. Over time a diet low in calcium can increase the risk of developing brittle bone disease (osteoporosis). One of the easiest ways to meet your daily calcium requirement is to consume two or three portions of milk, yoghurt or cheese. It's easy. All you need is:

- ❑ 200 ml (7 fl oz) glass of semi-skimmed or skimmed milk—plain or flavoured
- ❑ 150 gram (5½ oz) pot of low fat natural or fruit yogurt
- ❑ 30 gram (1 oz) match-box-sized piece of cheese

For more information go to www.milk.co.uk

Cheese – a great source of calcium

Perfect for sandwich fillings, snacks and toppings for pasta and with gratin dishes, cheese also contributes a fair number of calories. Most cheese is around 30 per cent fat, much of it saturated.

Ricotta and cottage cheese are good low fat choices – usually less than 7 per cent fat. Use them as an alternative to butter or margarine for sandwiches. It's worth trying fresh ricotta from a deli – you may find its soft creamy texture and fresh flavour tastier than pre-packaged tub ricotta. When making lasagne, use creamy ricotta instead of white sauce. Flavoured cottage cheese or natural cottage cheese with freshly snipped chives or basil and a twist of black pepper make ideal low fat toppings for toast and crackers for snacks and light lunches.

Although there are a number of good reduced fat cheeses available, others can lose out in the flavour stakes for a relatively small reduction in fat. If you are a real cheese lover and having a hard time finding a tasty low fat one, try these tips for making the most of your higher fat cheese choices.

❑ Consider eating a little of a strong-flavoured cheese rather than a lot of something bland and tasteless.
❑ Shave a few strips of fresh Parmesan over pasta – a vegetable peeler does the job nicely. Grating and shaving helps a little cheese go a long way.
❑ Enjoy full fat cheeses in small amounts occasionally. This includes regular types of cheddar, blue vein, Swiss, brie, Camembert, gouda and havarti.
❑ Try some mozzarella cheese – whole milk or semi-skimmed – it may contain less fat than some reduced fat cheeses. Grate and sprinkle over stuffed vegetables such as aubergines or peppers, baked potatoes and pizzas before cooking.

CHOCOLATE MILK

GI 24 (low fat, sweetened with aspartame)
GI 34 (low fat, sweetened with sugar)

Flavoured milks are available in regular or low fat varieties with relatively modest amounts of added sugar (about 4 per cent) compared with soft drinks (11–12 per cent). Adding a moderate amount of sugar in the form of chocolate syrup or powder or other flavours does not significantly raise the GI of low fat milk. For many people, children and adults alike, who don't like the taste of plain milk or prefer something sweeter, this dairy choice can add some extra vitamins and minerals to the day's nutrient intake. However, the choice of a low fat type is important, as is a smaller, rather than larger, serve size if you're watching your calorie intake.

Although some parents might be concerned that flavoured milk simply adds extra sugar to their child's diet, it is a far more nutritious drink than a soft drink. A study in Canada has shown that children and teenagers who drink flavoured milk consume fewer soft drinks and fewer fruit drinks than those who do not, and have far better calcium intakes. This is significant when you consider that maximum bone strength is built up in our younger years and 82 per cent of our children aren't getting the recommended three daily serves of dairy foods they need.

Serving suggestions

- Make flavoured milk ice-cubes for snacks after school or on hot days.
- Blend flavoured milk with fruit and a dollop of low fat yoghurt for a quick smoothie.

CUSTARD

GI 43 (made with powder)

Custard is a good source of calcium and protein, especially for young children who don't like drinking milk. Packet custard based on wheat starch is quick and easy to prepare. Make it with semi-skimmed milk or low fat calcium-enriched soya milk and sprinkle a little freshly grated nutmeg on top for that traditional 'baked custard' look. Serve hot or cold with fresh or canned fruit – especially peaches or nectarines – or with a sliced banana stirred through.

Serving suggestions

- Refuel with a chilled single-serve pot of custard from the dairy dessert cabinet in the supermarket. Look for low fat varieties.
- Top winter warming desserts like apple and rhubarb crumble with a creamy custard sauce or use as a filling for pastries.
- For that special occasion, make a 'real' custard with milk, a vanilla pod and egg. Bring 500 ml (17 fl oz) of milk almost to the boil, remove from the heat, add a vanilla pod and set aside for 15 minutes to infuse. Meanwhile, whisk 5 egg yolks and 125 grams (4½ oz) of caster sugar in a bowl until thick and creamy. Remove the vanilla pod from the milk and pour the milk into the egg mixture, stirring vigorously. Place in a heavy-based saucepan and cook over a medium heat (do not allow to boil), stirring constantly, until the custard thickens. Strain if the custard becomes lumpy.

DAIRY DESSERTS

GI 32–48 (chilled, low fat)

From flavoured crème fraîche to mousse, rice pudding to tiramisu, today's refrigerated dairy cabinet is filled with tempting, ready-to-eat, light, creamy, even aerated, desserts packed in single-serve pots, packs and pouches. Without the effort needed to whip up a pudding from scratch, they provide a guilt-free after-dinner indulgence or a convenient snack on the run and without adding too many calories. Because they are milk based they can be a useful source of calcium and provide an alternative to yoghurt or ice-cream when you want something sweet. Choose low fat, low GI products and enjoy in moderation.

Serving suggestions

- Lightly grill fresh fruits and serve topped with a dollop of a chocolate or vanilla dairy dessert as an alternative to ice-cream or yoghurt.
- Enjoy single-serve dairy desserts as a satisfying snack when you need to refuel on the run or as an alternative to other morning or afternoon snacks.

FLAVOURED MILK POWDERS

GI 40 (Milo® made with semi-skimmed milk)

Milk is an important source of calcium throughout life. Adding a moderate amount of refined sugar in the form of Milo®, Ovaltine® or Horlicks® does not significantly raise the GI of semi-skimmed or skimmed milk. As with flavoured milks from the chilled dairy cabinet, this is an excellent dairy choice for children and adults that can help add some extra vitamins and minerals to the day's nutrient intake.

ICE-CREAM

GI 37–49 (low fat)

Ice-cream is not just a treat, it's a useful source of bone-building calcium plus some protein and the other essential vitamins and minerals found in milk. Because it contains added sugar, the GI generally tends to be a little higher than milk and yoghurt. Look for low fat varieties when you shop – you'll find that some taste as good if not better than their full fat counterparts. Add a scoop to milkshakes and smoothies and enjoy a small portion as a snack or dessert with fruit.

Serving suggestions

For a satisfying snack or quick breakfast in a glass, whip up a nutritious smoothie. Start with your fruit combination and add about 250 ml (9 fl oz) of milk and a scoop of low fat ice-cream or yoghurt to make it creamy. Boost the vitamin and fibre content with a little wheat germ or bran. For a thicker texture, blend with frozen fruit. If you don't have time to freeze the fruit, simply whirl in some crushed ice until the smoothie is as thick as you like. Here are some combinations to try:

- Tangy banana and apple – blend until smooth: 1 frozen banana, 125 ml (4 fl oz) of orange juice, 1 gala apple, peeled and roughly cut into chunks, 125 ml (4 fl oz) of semi-skimmed milk and a scoop of low fat ice-cream or yoghurt.
- Raspberry and peach – blend until smooth: 125 ml (4 fl oz) of apple juice, 2 scoops of low fat ice-cream, 1 peeled, sliced and partially frozen peach and 6 or 7 partially frozen raspberries. Whirl in a few spoonfuls of crushed ice and serve.
- Creamy banana and strawberry – blend until smooth: 1 banana, 6 strawberries, sliced, 250 ml (9 fl oz) of semi-skimmed milk and 1 scoop of low fat ice-cream. Whirl in a few spoonfuls of crushed ice and serve.

INSTANT PUDDINGS
GI 40–47

Instant puddings, like custard, are useful in helping children and teenagers (and adults) achieve the three servings of dairy foods a day they need to build strong bones. These dried packet mixes come in a range of flavours and are the speediest way to whip up a nutritious, satisfying and economical dessert and because they are so easy to make, even young children can help in the kitchen. Choose low fat milk or low fat calcium-enriched soya milk for these dairy desserts and serve with fresh or canned fruit.

Serving suggestions

- Make instant pudding iced treats for after-school snacks. Combine pudding and milk in a deep bowl and beat with a mixer following the packet instructions. Spoon the mixture into individual cupcake containers and leave to set for about a minute. Insert ice-cream sticks into the centre and freeze.
- Whip up banana smoothies with extra flavour by blending a tablespoon of instant pudding mix per 250 ml (9 fl oz) of milk.

MILK

GI 27–34 (range of skimmed to regular fat milks)

Nutritionally, milk packs a punch. It's long been valued for protein, the bone-building minerals calcium and phosphorus and vitamins such as riboflavin (vitamin B2). Milk also has a low GI – a combination of the moderate glycaemic effect of its sugar (lactose) plus the milk protein, which forms a soft curd in the stomach and slows down the rate of stomach emptying. Regular whole milk is high in saturated fat, but these days there is a wide range of milk to suit everybody's needs, including semi-skimmed or skimmed varieties. So enjoy a glass of milk or a milkshake or smoothie and use milk in your cooking for desserts and sauces, but opt for the semi-skimmed and skimmed types.

We sometimes include buttermilk in our recipes. Despite its name, buttermilk isn't high in fat – it's made from skimmed milk. Specially chosen bacterial cultures are added in its manufacture to give the traditional texture and slightly sour taste that makes it popular for baking.

Serving suggestions

- Hot milk and honey makes a nutritious nightcap. Research shows that people do sleep more soundly after a warm milk drink at night. Warming the milk activates an amino acid called tryptophan, which the body converts to serotonin, the hormone associated with calmness and wellbeing.
- When you're out for a coffee choose a skimmed milk café latte (a 'skinny latte') or cappuccino and get a calcium boost!
- White sauce is used in dishes such as mornay, lasagne and savoury soufflés and is the base for many sauces. To make it, the traditional method is to melt 2 tablespoons of butter or margarine in a small saucepan over a low heat. Blend in 2 tablespoons of plain flour and cook over a low heat for 1–2 minutes, then slowly add 250 ml (9 fl oz) of milk, stirring constantly until smooth and thickened. Season to taste with salt and freshly ground black pepper, celery salt, nutmeg, or a few tablespoons of chopped chives or parsley. You can make a lower fat version by heating 250 ml (9 fl oz) of semi-skimmed milk with 1 whole peeled onion and a bay leaf. When hot, stir in 1 tablespoon of cornflour blended with a little cold milk and stir over a low heat until thickened. Remove the onion and bay leaf and discard and season as above.

SOYA MILK
GI 36–44 (reduced fat, calcium fortified)
Drinking this completely dairy- and lactose-free beverage is an easy way to include soya protein in your diet. Whole soyabeans – which are usually GM/GE free (check the label)

– are mixed with filtered water and flavourings to produce a milk-like product. Once enjoyed by vegetarians, soya milk has become increasing popular, possibly because it tastes good and is recognised to be rich in phytoestrogens, nutrients that are known to have health benefits.

Soya milk is available fresh from the chilled dairy cabinet, in long life packs and in powdered forms. You can also buy flavoured products. To ensure it is a suitable alternative to regular dairy milk, soya milk is often enriched with a range of vitamins and minerals including calcium and riboflavin (vitamin B12). Choose a low fat, calcium-enriched milk and use it exactly as you would regular milk – on your breakfast cereal, with hot or cold drinks or in your cooking when making desserts and sauces.

Serving suggestions

If you haven't tried calcium-enriched, low fat soya milk before, here are some easy ways to get started.

- Mix it in with mashed sweet potato, pumpkin or potato; or in a combination of all three vegetables.
- Try a soya latte or soya banana smoothie or use in other flavoured milk drinks.
- Use it to make white sauce for lasagne or moussaka.
- Make dairy desserts with soya milk.

SOYA YOGHURT

GI 50 (fruit flavoured, sweetened with sugar)

Soya yoghurt is usually made from soyabeans or soya protein rather than soya milk. Look for calcium-enriched, low fat varieties and use in exactly the same way as you would dairy yoghurts as a snack or dessert, or added to smoothies and shakes. Unflavoured soya yoghurt can be used in dips, sauces and spreads.

YOGHURT

GI range 14–43
GI 14–21 (low fat, flavoured, no added sugar)
GI 26–43 (low fat, flavoured, sweetened with sugar)

Yoghurt is a concentrated milk product rich in calcium, riboflavin and protein, and all varieties have low GI values, mainly due to the combination of acidity and high protein. Artificially sweetened, flavoured yoghurts have the lowest GI values and contain fewer calories than the naturally sweetened flavoured versions. Drinking yoghurts are also available and will have similar GI values. Low fat yoghurt provides the most calcium for the least calories (520 mg calcium in a 200 gram/7 oz pot).

People who are lactose intolerant can usually safely consume yoghurt without experiencing abdominal distress. Special types of bacteria added to some yoghurts (eg. Bifidobacteria) may colonise the large intestine and provide health benefits. Research in this area is still controversial.

Eating a 200 gram (7 oz) pot of yoghurt is equivalent to drinking a 250 ml (9 fl oz) glass of milk. As with other dairy products, choose the low fat varieties and enjoy throughout the day with breakfast cereals or as a snack or dessert.

Serving suggestions

Always keep a pot of low fat plain yoghurt in the fridge, trying different brands until you find one you like. It's a great base for dips, salad dressings and sauces – sweet and savoury.

- Serve chicken salad with a yoghurt dressing made from a 200 gram (7 oz) pot of low fat plain yoghurt, 2 tablespoons of lemon juice, a couple of teaspoons of a tangy mango chutney and 2 tablespoons of finely chopped mint.
- Spice plain yoghurt with a little ground cumin and

cardamom to make a sauce for topping burgers or falafel rolls. Add fresh mint for a finishing touch.

- Make a spicy Indian 'lassi' drink by blending 200 grams (7 oz) of low fat natural yoghurt with ½ teaspoon of ground cumin and a pinch of salt to taste. Chill. Just before serving, stir in 1/4 teaspoon of finely minced onion and a few strips of finely sliced green chilli. Pour into a tall glass over lots of ice-cubes and serve – delicious as an appetiser before an Indian meal.

- For a sweeter taste, mango lassis are a meal in a glass or a delicious way to finish a spicy dinner. You can make this lassi in about 5 minutes by combining in a blender 1 medium sized mango, diced, with 125 ml (4 fl oz) of freshly squeezed orange juice, a few spoonfuls of ice-cubes, 1 tablespoon of pure floral honey or a little more to taste, and 1 teaspoon of rosewater if you have it. Process for about 30 seconds until the ingredients are just blended. Add 300 grams (10½ oz) of low fat natural yoghurt and whizz for another 30–40 seconds until it's frothy. Makes 4 glasses (250 ml/9 fl oz each).

low gi eating made easy
Tables

Here's your easy and reliable reference to the GI of foods. Use these tables to choose the best carbs for your health and to enjoy low GI foods every meal, every day.

Remember, it is carb quality that counts.

We have categorised the foods A to Z under the following headings:

- Bakery products – including cakes and muffins
- Beans, peas and lentils – including split peas, lentils, chickpeas and baked beans
- Beverages – including fruit and vegetable juices, soft drinks, flavoured milk and sport drinks
- Biscuits – including commercial sweet biscuits, savoury crispbreads and plain crackers
- Bread – including sliced white and wholemeal bread, fruit breads and flat breads
- Breakfast cereals – including processed cereals, muesli, oats and porridge
- Cereal grains – including couscous, bulghur and barley
- Dairy products and alternatives – including milk, yoghurt, ice-creams, dairy desserts and soya products
- Fruits – including fresh, canned and dried fruit
- Miscellaneous – including various fast foods
- Pasta, noodles and rice
- Snack foods – including muesli bars, fruit sticks and straps and nuts
- Sweeteners and spreads – including sugars, honey and jam
- Vegetables – including green vegetables, salad vegetables, root vegetables and soups

All you need to do for everyday low GI eating is make **MOST** of your carbohydrate choices from the **EVERYDAY** foods, taking into account the serving sizes shown. Remember larger servings will increase the glycaemic load of the food and may change its ranking.

Note: We have organised the **EVERYDAY** foods into those you can eat according to your appetite and those where you need to exercise a bit of restraint and some sensible portion caution.

EVERYDAY foods

These 'eat according to your appetite' foods have a **low GI** and a **low GL** (depending on how much you put on your plate). They are slowly digested, long-lasting foods, which are the best sources of sustained energy. Their low GI gives them a high fill-up factor which means you can eat them according to appetite. Some of your EVERYDAY foods – granary bread, fresh fruit, low fat yoghurt, split peas, soya beans, rolled oats, pure floral honey and sour-dough bread.

EVERYDAY CAUTION WITH PORTION foods

These foods have a moderate or low GI and a moderate to high GL, again, depending on your serving size. They're great sources of carbohydrate but it's sensible to give some thought to the quantity of these foods, because of their potential to have a high GL if you overload your plate or go back for seconds or thirds. Some of your **EVERYDAY CAUTION WITH PORTION** foods – fruit juices, noodles, pasta, rice, soft drinks, crumpets, flavoured milks, fruit breads, muesli bars and sultanas.

OCCASIONAL foods

These foods have high GI values but a moderate GL. Their high GI makes them rapidly digested and much less satisfying than the **EVERYDAY** foods so keep them occasional. Some foods that are higher in saturated fat have also been included in this group. Some of your **OCCASIONAL** foods – potatoes, scones, crackers and processed cereals.

KEEP FOR A TREAT foods

These are high GI and high GL or are high in saturated fat. Many of them are standard fare in our British diet but by stimulating blood glucose and insulin spikes they contribute to our risk of obesity, diabetes and heart disease. Don't be fooled by the low fat nature of some of them! Some of your **KEEP FOR A TREAT** foods – puffed cereals, white bread, bagels, jelly beans, chocolate.

BAKERY PRODUCTS			
Everyday foods	Everyday caution with portion foods	Occasional foods	Keep for a treat foods
	Apple muffin, home-made 60 g	Angel food cake, plain 50 g	Banana cake, home-made 80 g
		Bran muffin, commercially made 125 g	Blueberry muffin, commercially made 125 g
		Carrot cake, commercially made 125 g	Chocolate cake, made from packet mix with icing 125 g
		Crumpet, white 50 g	Croissant, plain 60 g
		Scones, plain, made from packet mix 50 g	Cupcake, strawberry-iced 38 g
		Sponge cake, plain, unfilled 63 g	Pound cake, plain 50 g
			Vanilla cake made from packet mix with vanilla icing 125 g

BEANS, PEAS AND LENTILS

Everyday foods	Everyday caution with portion foods	Occasional foods	Keep for a treat foods
Baked beans, canned in tomato sauce 150 g	Black-eyed beans, soaked, boiled 150 g		
Black beans, boiled 150 g	Broad beans 80 g		
Borlotti beans, canned, drained 75 g	Haricot beans, cooked, canned 150 g		
Butter beans, canned, drained 75 g	Kidney beans, red, canned, drained 150 g		
Butter beans, dried, boiled 150 g			
Cannellini beans 85 g			
Chickpeas, canned in brine 150 g			
Chickpeas, dried, boiled 150 g			
Dark red kidney beans, canned, drained 150 g			
Four bean mix, canned, drained 75 g			
Green lentils, canned 50 g			

BEANS, PEAS AND LENTILS			
Everyday foods	**Everyday caution with portion foods**	**Occasional foods**	**Keep for a treat foods**
Green lentils, dried, boiled 150 g			
Haricot beans, dried, boiled 150 g			
Kidney beans, red, dried, boiled 150 g			
Lima beans, baby, frozen, reheated 150 g			
Mung beans 150 g			
Peas, dried, boiled 150 g			
Red lentils, dried, boiled 150 g			
Soyabeans, canned, drained 150 g			
Soyabeans, dried, boiled 150 g			
Split peas, yellow, boiled 20 mins 150 g			

BEVERAGES

Everyday foods	Everyday caution with portion foods	Occasional foods	Keep for a treat foods
Carrot juice, freshly made 250 ml	Apple juice, no added sugar 250 ml	Isostar® sports drink 250 ml	Milo® powder in full fat milk 250 ml
Coffee, black, no milk or sugar 200 ml	Coca-Cola®, soft drink 250 ml	Lucozade®, original, sparkling glucose drink 250 ml	
Diet soft drinks 250 ml	Cranberry Juice Cocktail, Ocean Spray 250 ml		
Milo® powder in skimmed or reduced fat milk 250 ml	Fanta®, orange soft drink 250 ml		
Tomato juice, no added sugar 250 ml	Grapefruit juice, unsweetened 250 ml		
	Orange juice, unsweetened 250 ml		
	Pineapple juice, unsweetened 250 ml		

BISCUITS			
Everyday foods	**Everyday caution with portion foods**	**Occasional foods**	**Keep for a treat foods**
Ryvita® crispbread 25 g		Crispbread, generic 25 g	
		Crispbread, gluten-free 21 g	
		Digestive biscuits, plain 25 g	
		Oatcakes 55 g	
		Rice cakes, puffed, white 25 g	
		Wafer biscuits, vanilla, plain 25 g	
		Water crackers, plain 25 g	

BREAD

Everyday foods	Everyday caution with portion foods	Occasional foods	Keep for a treat foods
Fruit & Muesli loaf, Bürgen® 40 g	Gluten-free low carbohydrate 30 g	Bun, hamburger, white 53 g	Bagel, white 70 g
Fruit Loaf, thick sliced 30 g	Gluten-free multigrain brown, sliced 30 g	Dark rye bread 30 g	Baguette, white 30 g
Pumpernickel bread 30 g	Gluten-free mutigrain white, sliced 30 g	Gluten-free bread, white, sliced 30 g	Light rye bread 30 g
Rye bread, Bürgen® 40 g	Hibran, Bürgen 44 g	Stuffing, bread 30 g	Melba toast, plain 30 g
Sourdough bread, organic, stoneground, wholemeal 32 g	Multigrain sandwich bread 30 g	Sunflower Maltigrain, Allinson 47 g	
Sourdough rye bread 30 g	Pitta bread, white 75 g	White bread, regular sliced 30 g	
Sourdough wheat bread 30 g	Tasty wholemeal, Kingsmill 38 g		
Soya and Linseed, Bürgen 40 g			

BREAKFAST CEREALS			
Everyday foods	**Everyday caution with portion foods**	**Occasional foods**	**Keep for a treat foods**
All-Bran®, Kellogg's® 30 g	Frosties®, Kellogg's® 30 g	Bran Flakes, Kellogg's® 30 g	Rice Krispies®, Kellogg's® 30 g
Oat bran, raw, unprocessed 10 g	Muesli, Natural 45 g	Cornflakes, Crunchy Nut, Kellogg's® 30 g	
Porridge, regular, made from oats with water 30 g	Special K®, regular, Kellogg's® 30 g	Cornflakes®, Kellogg's® 30 g	
Rolled Oats, raw 30 g		Porridge, instant, made with water 30 g	
		Puffed Wheat breakfast cereal 30 g	
		Shredded Wheat 30 g	
		Sultana Bran, Kellogg's® 30 g	

CEREAL GRAINS

Everyday foods	Everyday caution with portion foods	Occasional foods	Keep for a treat foods
Barley, pearl, boiled 150 g	Barley, rolled, raw 50 g		
Semolina, cooked 150 g	Buckwheat, boiled 150 g		
	Cornmeal (polenta), boiled 150 g		
	Couscous, boiled 5 mins 150 g		
	Quinoa, organic, raw, 50 g		
	Rye, raw 50 g		
	Wheat, cracked, bulghur, ready to eat 150 g		
	Whole-wheat kernels, raw 50 g		

DAIRY PRODUCTS – ICE-CREAM, CUSTARD AND DESSERTS

Everyday foods	Everyday caution with portion foods	Occasional foods	Keep for a treat foods
Custard, vanilla, reduced fat 100 ml			Custard, home-made from milk, wheat starch and sugar 100 ml
			Ice Cream, Regular, full fat, average of several types 50 g

DAIRY PRODUCTS – MILK AND ALTERNATIVES			
Everyday foods	**Everyday caution with portion foods**	**Occasional foods**	**Keep for a treat foods**
Milk, semi-skimmed, low fat (1.4%) 250ml			Milk (3.6% fat) 250 ml
Skimmed milk, low fat (0.1%) 250 ml			
Soya milk, full fat (3%) 250 ml			
Soya milk, low fat, calcium-fortified 250 ml			

DAIRY PRODUCTS – YOGHURT			
Everyday foods	**Everyday caution with portion foods**	**Occasional foods**	**Keep for a treat foods**
Yoghurt, Ski™, low fat, with sugar, strawberry 200 g Yoghurt, Ski™, no fat, with sugar, all flavours 200 g	Soya yoghurt, 2% fat, with sugar, peach and mango 200 g		

FRUIT FRESH

Everyday foods	Everyday caution with portion foods	Occasional foods	Keep for a treat foods
Apple, fresh 120 g	Banana, raw 120 g		
Apricots, fresh 168 g	Watermelon, raw 120 g		
Avocado 120 g			
Cantaloupe, fresh 120 g			
Cherries, dark, raw 120 g			
Custard apple, fresh, flesh only 120 g			
Figs 50 g			
Grapefruit, fresh 120 g			
Grapes, fresh 120 g			
Kiwi fruit, fresh 120 g			
Lemon 40 g			
Lime 40 g			
Mango, fresh 120 g			
Orange, fresh 120 g			
Papaya (pawpaw), fresh 120 g			
Peach, fresh 120 g			
Pear, fresh 120 g			
Pineapple, fresh 120 g			
Plum, raw 120 g			
Raspberries 65 g			
Strawberries, fresh 120 g			

FRUIT – CANNED			
Everyday foods	**Everyday caution with portion foods**	**Occasional foods**	**Keep for a treat foods**
Peaches, canned, in heavy syrup 120 g	Apricots, canned in light syrup 120 g	Lychees, canned, in syrup, drained 120 g	
Peaches, canned, in light syrup 120 g			
Peaches, canned, in natural juice 120 g			
Pear halves, canned, in natural juice 120 g			
Pear halves, canned, in reduced-sugar syrup 120 g			

FRUIT – DRIED			
Everyday foods	**Everyday caution with portion foods**	**Occasional foods**	**Keep for a treat foods**
Apple, dried 60 g Apricots, dried 60 g Prunes, pitted 60 g	Cranberries, dried, sweetened 40 g Dates, Arabic, dried, vacuum-packed 55 g Figs, dried, tenderised 60 g Raisins 60 g Sultanas 60 g		

MISCELLANEOUS – FAST FOOD

Everyday foods	Everyday caution with portion foods	Occasional foods	Keep for a treat foods
Consommé, clear, chicken or vegetable 250 ml	Black bean soup, canned 250 ml		Chicken nuggets, frozen reheated in microwave 5 mins, 100 g
Lentil soup, canned 250 ml	Chicken Tikka Biryani 450 g		Pizza, Super Supreme, pan, Pizza Hut 130 g
Minestrone soup, Traditional, canned 250 ml	Chicken Tikka Masala & Pilau Rice, Be Good To Yourself range 400 g		Pizza, Super Supreme, thin and crispy, Pizza Hut 100 g
Tomato soup, canned 250 ml	Fish fingers 100 g		
	Green pea soup, canned 250 ml		
	Lamb Bhuna & Rice, 500 g		
	Split pea soup, canned 250 ml		
	Sushi, salmon 100 g		

PASTA

Everyday foods	Everyday caution with portion foods	Occasional foods	Keep for a treat foods
	2 Minute noodles, 99% fat free, Maggi 80 g		2 Minute noodles, regular, Maggi 80 g
	Capellini pasta, white boiled 180 g		Rice pasta, brown, boiled 180 g
	Fettuccine, egg, boiled 180 g		
	Gnocchi, cooked 180 g		
	Linguine pasta, thick, durum wheat, boiled 180 g		
	Linguine pasta, thin, durum wheat, boiled 180 g		
	Macaroni, white, durum wheat, boiled 180 g		
	Mung bean noodles (bean thread), dried, boiled 180 g		
	Ravioli, meat-filled, durum wheat flour, boiled 180 g		
	Rice noodles, dried, boiled 180 g		

Everyday foods	Everyday caution with portion foods	Occasional foods	Keep for a treat foods
	PASTA		
	Rice noodles, fresh, boiled 180 g		
	Rice vermicelli, dried, boiled, Chinese 180 g		
	Soba noodles, instant, served in soup 180 g		
	Spaghetti, white, durum wheat 180 g		
	Spaghetti, whole-meal, boiled 180 g		
	Spirali pasta, white, durum wheat 180 g		
	Tortellini, cheese, boiled 180 g		
	Udon noodles, plain 180 g		
	Vermicelli, white, durum wheat, boiled 180 g		

RICE			
Everyday foods	**Everyday caution with portion foods**	**Occasional foods**	**Keep for a treat foods**
	Basmati rice, white, boiled 150 g		Instant rice, white, cooked 6 mins with water 150 g
	Wild rice, boiled 150 g		Jasmine rice, white, long-grain, cooked in rice cooker 150 g
			Risotto rice, Arborio, boiled 150 g

SNACK FOODS

Everyday foods	Everyday caution with portion foods	Occasional foods	Keep for a treat foods
Jelly, diet, made from crystals with water 125 g	Cashew nuts 30 g Marshmallows, plain, pink and white 25 g Muesli bar, chewy, with choc chips or fruit 31 g Muesli bar, crunchy, with dried fruit 30 g Peanuts, roasted, 50 g Pecan nuts, raw 50 g Popcorn, plain, cooked in microwave 20 g Taco shells, cornmeal-based, baked 40 g	M&M's®, peanut 30 g Pretzels, oven-baked, traditional wheat flavour 30 g	Cadbury's® Milk Chocolate, plain 30 g Chocolate, Milk, plain, Nestlé® 50 g Chocolate, Milk, white, Nestlé® 50 g Corn chips, plain, salted 50 g Dark chocolate, plain, regular 30 g Jelly beans 30 g Licorice, soft 60 g Mars Bar®, regular 60 g Milky Bar®, plain white chocolate, Nestlé® 50 g Polos®, peppermint 30 g Pop-Tarts™, chocotastic 50 g Skittles® 50 g Twix® bar 60 g

SWEETENERS AND SPREADS			
Everyday foods	**Everyday caution with portion foods**	**Occasional foods**	**Keep for a treat foods**
Honey, pure floral (various) 25 g	Glucose tablets 10 g		
Hummous, regular 30 g	Honey, blended, various 25 g		
Jam, strawberry, regular 30 g	Marmalade, orange 30 g		
Maple syrup, pure, Canadian 24 g	Sugar 20 g		
Nutella®, hazelnut spread 20 g			

VEGETABLES

Everyday foods	Everyday caution with portion foods	Occasional foods	Keep for a treat foods
Alfalfa sprouts 6 g	New potato, canned 150 g	Desiree potato, peeled, boiled 150 g	French fries, frozen, reheated in microwave 150 g
Artichokes, globe, fresh or canned in brine 80 g	Pumpkin 80 g	Instant mashed potato 150 g	
Asparagus 100 g	Swede, cooked 150 g	New potato, unpeeled and boiled 150 g	
Aubergine 100 g	Sweet potato, baked 150 g	Parsnips 80 g	
Bean sprouts, raw 14 g	Yam, peeled, boiled 150 g		
Beetroot, canned 80 g			
Bok choi 100 g			
Broccoli 60 g			
Brussel sprouts 100 g			
Cabbage 70 g			
Carrots, peeled, boiled 80 g			
Cauliflower 60 g			
Celery 40 g			
Courgette 100 g			
Cucumber 45 g			
Endive 30 g			
Fennel 90 g			
Green beans 70 g			
Leeks 80 g			
Lettuce 50 g			

VEGETABLES			
Everyday foods	**Everyday caution with portion foods**	**Occasional foods**	**Keep for a treat foods**
Mangetout sprouts 15 g			
Mushrooms 35 g			
Onions, 30 g			
Peas, green, frozen, boiled 80 g			
Pepper 80 g			
Radishes 15 g			
Rhubarb 125 g			
Rocket 30 g			
Shallots 10 g			
Spinach 75 g			
Squash, yellow 70 g			
Sweetcorn, on the cob, boiled 80 g			
Sweetcorn, whole kernel, canned, drained 80 g			
Taro 150 g			
Tomato 150 g			
Turnip 120 g			
Watercress 8 g			

Acknowledgements

In thanking colleagues who have helped us with this book, we would like to single out Hachette Livre's Publishing and Production Director, Fiona Hazard, for making it all 'so easy', our editor, Jacquie Brown, for her attention to detail and eye for consistency and our project editor Anna Waddington for whom nothing is too much trouble.

We wanted to create special Low GI Eating Made Easy tables to make it really easy for readers to choose healthy low GI foods, and we could not have done so without the cheerful efforts and database wizardry of Associate Prof Gareth Denyer at the University of Sydney.

We would also like to thank Johanna Burani whose suggestions for the US edition of The Top 100 Foods we have incorporated into this book and for permission to include her Cherry Oat Crunchies recipe from Good Carbs, Bad Carbs (Marlowe & Company); Kate Marsh who checked the information on PCOS for us and dietitian, Penny Hunking, who has helped us with this UK edition.

Further Resources

For further information on GI

www.glycemicindex.com
This is the University of Sydney's glycemic index website where you can learn about GI and access the GI database which includes the most up-to-date listing of the GI of foods that have been published in international scientific journals.

http://ginews.blogspot.com
GI News is the official glycemic index newsletter published online each month by the University of Sydney's GI Group.

www.gisymbol.com.au
The Glycemic Index (GI) Symbol Program is a food labelling program with strict nutritional criteria that aims to help people make informed food choices. The site includes a complete listing of foods carrying the GI symbol.

For information on:

Food labelling and food additives

Food Standards Agency
www.food.gov.uk

Finding a dietitian

British Dietetic Association (BDA)
www.bda.uk.com

Diabetes

Diabetes UK

www.diabetesuk.co.uk

Heart health

Heart UK

www.heartuk.org.uk

British Heart Foundation

www.bhf.org.uk

PCOS

The main resource for women with PCOS in the UK

www.verity-pcos.org.uk

Information source for polycystic ovarian syndrome (PCOS), diabetes and insulin resistance.

www.diagnosemefirst.com

Index

About the authors

Kaye Foster-Powell is an accredited practising dietitian with extensive experience in diabetes management: she provides consultancy on all aspects of the glycaemic index.

Jennie Brand-Miller is an internationally recognised authority on carbohydrates and health. She is Professor of Human Nutrition at the University of Sydney and President of the Nutrition Society of Australia.

Jennie and Kaye have co-authored 16 books in the worldwide bestselling New Glucose Revolution series, which has sold over three million copies and is changing the way the world views carbohydrates.

Philippa Sandall is an editor and writer who specialises in food, nutrition, health and lifesytle. She was closely involved in creating the first New Glucose Revolution title with Jennie and Kays in 1995, *The GI Factor*, and has played an integral role in developing and managing the series.